Geriatric Anesthesia

Editors

CHARLES H. BROWN IV
MARK D. NEUMAN

ANESTHESIOLOGY CLINICS

www.anesthesiology.theclinics.com

Consulting Editor
LEE A. FLEISHER

September 2015 • Volume 33 • Number 3

ELSEVIER

1600 John F. Kennedy Boulevard • Suite 1800 • Philadelphia, Pennsylvania, 19103-2899
http://www.theclinics.com

ANESTHESIOLOGY CLINICS Volume 33, Number 3
September 2015 ISSN 1932-2275, ISBN-13: 978-0-323-39551-9

Editor: Patrick Manley
Developmental Editor: Kristen Helm

Anesthesiology Clinics (ISSN 1932-2275) is published quarterly by Elsevier Inc., 360 Park Avenue South, New York, NY 10010-1710. Months of issue are March, June, September, and December. Periodicals postage paid at New York, NY and at additional mailing offices. Subscription prices are $160.00 per year (US student/resident), $330.00 per year (US individuals), $400.00 per year (Canadian individuals), $533.00 per year (US institutions), $674.00 per year (Canadian institutions), $225.00 per year (Canadian and foreign student/resident), $455.00 per year (foreign individuals), and $674.00 per year (foreign institutions). To receive student and resident rate, orders must be accompanied by name of affiliated institution, date of term, and the *signature* of program/residency coordinator on institutions letterhead. Orders will be billed at individual rate until proof of status is received. Foreign air speed delivery is included in all *Clinics'* subscription prices. All prices are subject to change without notice. POSTMASTER: Send address changes to *Anesthesiology Clinics,* Elsevier Health Sciences Division, Subscription Customer Service, 3251 Riverport Lane, Maryland Heights, MO 63043. Customer Service (orders, claims, online, change of address): Elsevier Health Sciences Division, Subscription Customer Service, 3251 Riverport Lane, Maryland Heights, MO 63043. **Tel:1-800-654-2452 (U.S. and Canada); 314-447-8871 (outside U.S. and Canada). Fax: 314-447-8029. E-mail: journalscustomerservice-usa@elsevier. com (for print support); journalsonlinesupport-usa@elsevier.com (for online support).**

Reprints. For copies of 100 or more of articles in this publication, please contact the Commercial Reprints Department, Elsevier Inc., 360 Park Avenue South, New York, NY 10010-1710. Tel.: 212-633-3874; Fax: 212-633-3820; E-mail: reprints@elsevier.com.

Anesthesiology Clinics, is also published in Spanish by McGraw-Hill Inter-americana Editores S. A., P.O. Box 5-237, 06500 Mexico D. F., Mexico.

Anesthesiology Clinics, is covered in *MEDLINE/PubMed (Index Medicus), Current Contents/Clinical Medicine, Excerpta Medica, ISI/BIOMED,* and *Chemical Abstracts.*

Contributors

CONSULTING EDITOR

LEE A. FLEISHER, MD, FACC, FAHA
Robert D. Dripps Professor and Chair of Anesthesiology and Critical Care, Professor of Medicine, Perelman School of Medicine at the University of Pennsylvania, Philadelphia, Pennsylvania

EDITORS

CHARLES H. BROWN IV, MD, MHS
Assistant Professor, Division of Cardiac Anesthesia, Department of Anesthesiology and Critical Care Medicine, Johns Hopkins School of Medicine, Baltimore, Maryland

MARK D. NEUMAN, MD, MSc
Assistant Professor, Department of Anesthesiology and Critical Care, Perelman School of Medicine at the University of Pennsylvania, Philadelphia, Pennsylvania

AUTHORS

SHAMSUDDIN AKHTAR, MD
Associate Professor of Anesthesiology and Pharmacology, Department of Anesthesiology, Yale University School of Medicine, New Haven, Connecticut

BRET D. ALVIS, MD
Assistant Professor of Anesthesiology and Critical Care Medicine, Division of Critical Care Medicine, Department of Anesthesiology, Vanderbilt University School of Medicine, Nashville, Tennessee

REBECCA A. ASLAKSON, MD, PhD
Associate Professor, Department of Anesthesiology and Critical Care Medicine, Palliative Medicine Program at the Kimmel Comprehensive Cancer Center at Johns Hopkins, The Johns Hopkins School of Medicine; Department of Health, Behavior, and Society, The Johns Hopkins Bloomberg School of Public Health, Baltimore, Maryland

RUBEN J. AZOCAR, MD
Tufts University School of Medicine, Boston, Massachusetts

MILES BERGER, MD, PhD
Assistant Professor, Neuroanesthesia Division, Department of Anesthesiology, Duke University Medical Center, Durham, North Carolina

MARK C. BICKET, MD
Clinical Fellow, Department of Anesthesia, Critical Care, and Pain Medicine, Massachusetts General Hospital, Harvard Medical School; Wang Ambulatory Care Center, Boston, Massachusetts

JEFFREY BROWNDYKE, PhD
Assistant Professor of Psychiatry and Behavioral Sciences, Division of Geriatric Behavioral Health, Duke University Medical Center, Durham, North Carolina

HARVEY JAY COHEN, MD
Walter Kempner Professor of Medicine and Director, Center for the Study of Aging and Human Development, Duke University Medical Center, Durham, North Carolina

JoANN COLEMAN, DNP, ACNP-BC
Coordinator, Department of Surgery, Sinai Center for Geriatric Surgery, Sinai Hospital, Baltimore, Maryland

STACIE G. DEINER, MD
Associate Professor, Departments of Anesthesiology, Neurosurgery, Geriatrics and Palliative Care, Icahn School of Medicine at Mount Sinai, New York, New York

ALLEN N. GUSTIN Jr, MD, FCCP
Associate Professor, Department of Anesthesiology, Stritch School of Medicine, Loyola University Medicine, Chicago, Illinois

CHRISTOPHER G. HUGHES, MD
Associate Professor of Anesthesiology and Critical Care Medicine, Division of Critical Care Medicine, Department of Anesthesiology, Vanderbilt University School of Medicine, Nashville, Tennessee

MAURICE F. JOYCE, MD, EdM
Clinical Associate, Department of Anesthesiology, Tufts Medical Center, Boston, Massachusetts

MARK R. KATLIC, MD, FACS
Chairman, Department of Surgery; Director, Sinai Center for Geriatric Surgery, Sinai Hospital, Baltimore, Maryland

LAEBEN LESTER, MD
Division of Cardiothoracic Anesthesia, Department of Anesthesiology and Critical Care Medicine, Johns Hopkins School of Medicine, Baltimore, Maryland

MICHAEL C. LEWIS, MBBS
University of Florida College of Medicine–Jacksonville, Jacksonville, Florida

JIANREN MAO, MD, PhD
Professor, Department of Anesthesia, Critical Care, and Pain Medicine, Massachusetts General Hospital, Harvard Medical School; Wang Ambulatory Care Center, Boston, Massachusetts

JOSEPH P. MATHEW, MD, MHSc, MBA
Jerry Reves Professor of Anesthesiology and Chairman, Department of Anesthesiology, Duke University Medical Center, Durham, North Carolina

JASON L. McKEOWN, MD
Department of Anesthesiology and Perioperative Medicine, University of Alabama, Birmingham, Birmingham, Alabama

MATTHEW T. MELLO, MD
University of Florida College of Medicine–Jacksonville, Jacksonville, Florida

JACOB W. NADLER, MD, PhD
Assistant Professor of Anesthesiology, University of Rochester Medical Center, Rochester, New York

MARIAM NAKHAIE, MD
Department of Anesthesiology, Tufts Medical Center, Boston, Massachusetts

VIKRAM PONNUSAMY, BA
Trinity College of Arts and Sciences, Duke University, Durham, North Carolina

RAMACHANDRAN RAMANI, MD
Associate Professor, Department of Anesthesiology, Yale University School of Medicine, New Haven, Connecticut

JOHN ADAM REICH, MD
Assistant Professor, Department of Anesthesiology, Tufts Medical Center, Boston, Massachusetts

G. ALEC ROOKE, MD, PhD
Professor, Department of Anesthesiology and Pain Medicine, University of Washington, Seattle, Washington

KATIE J. SCHENNING, MD, MPH
Assistant Professor, Department of Anesthesiology and Perioperative Medicine, Oregon Health and Science University, Portland, Oregon

NICCOLO TERRANDO, PhD
Assistant Professor, Basic Science Division, Department of Anesthesiology, Duke University Medical Center, Durham, North Carolina

ANDREA TSAI, MD
Department of Anesthesiology, Tufts Medical Center, Boston, Massachusetts

HEATHER E. WHITSON, MD, MHS
Associate Professor of Medicine (Geriatrics) and Ophthalmology, and Senior Fellow, Duke University Aging Center, Duke University Medical Center and Durham VA Geriatrics Research, Education, and Clinical Center (GRECC), Durham, North Carolina

SUSAN E. WOZNIAK, MD, MBA
Department of Surgery, Sinai Center for Geriatric Surgery, Sinai Hospital, Baltimore, Maryland

Contents

Creation of the American Society of Anesthesiologists Committee on Geriatric Anesthesia provided an opportunity for individuals to interact, strategize, and work with medical organizations outside of anesthesiology. These opportunities expanded with creation of the Society for the Advancement of Geriatric Anesthesia. The American Geriatrics Society provided a major boost when they realized it was important for surgical and related specialties to take an active role in the care of older patients. As a result, educational grants have improved residency training and established a major research grant program now managed by the National Institutes of Health. Nevertheless, for improved care of the older patient, the level of involvement has to increase.

An ever-changing health care system with a constantly increasing aging surgical population creates both opportunities for providing improved health care as well as significant challenges. Coordinated health care initiatives are needed if one is to adequately balance the need for evidence-based improved patient outcomes and the often-associated increased costs. In this article the authors postulate that a protocol-driven, multidisciplinary approach may be a pathway for implementing an effective triple aim to health care, especially in a frail geriatric population.

Physiology changes at the structural, functional, and molecular levels as people age, and every major organ system experiences physiologic change with time. The changes to the nervous system result mostly in cognitive impairments, the cardiovascular system develops higher blood pressures with lower cardiac output, the respiratory system undergoes a reduction of arterial oxyhemoglobin levels, the gastrointestinal system experiences delayed gastric emptying and reduction of hepatic metabolism, and the renal system experiences a diminished glomerular filtration rate. Combined, these changes create a complex physiologic condition. This unique physiology must be taken into consideration for geriatric patients undergoing general anesthesia.

Shamsuddin Akhtar and Ramachandran Ramani

Aging involves changes in several physiologic processes that lead to decreased volumes of distribution, slowed metabolism, and increased end-organ sensitivity to anesthetics. These changes generally result in increased potency. Elderly patients require less anesthetic medication, but the true extent of reduction is underappreciated and less uniformly practiced. The impact of potential anesthetic drug overdosing on intermediate and long-term outcomes is not fully appreciated. It may be necessary to consider age as a continuous variable for anesthetic drug dosing in older patients rather than treating adult versus elderly patients. Further pharmacologic studies are required in people more than 85 years old.

Mariam Nakhaie and Andrea Tsai

The preoperative assessment of geriatric patients provides an excellent opportunity to evaluate the patient for perioperative risk factors such as frailty, functional status, nutritional status, cardiovascular and pulmonary status, and substance dependence. It also provides an overall clinical picture on which health care providers can base a framework to reduce these risk factors.

Susan E. Wozniak, JoAnn Coleman, and Mark R. Katlic

The elderly preoperative patient benefits from an assessment that includes more than a routine physical examination and electrocardiogram. Such an assessment includes domains likely to affect the elderly: cognition, functionality, frailty, polypharmacy, nutrition, and social support. This fosters decisions based on functional age rather than chronologic age and on each patient as an individual. One such assessment is that promulgated by the American College of Surgeons National Surgery Quality Improvement Program/American Geriatrics Society Best Practice Guidelines. We should not miss any opportunity to improve results in this growing population of surgical patients.

Laeben Lester

The elderly population is growing. Geriatric patients undergo a large proportion of surgical procedures and have increased complications, morbidity, and mortality, which may be associated with increased intensive care unit time, length of stay, hospital readmission, and cost. Identification of optimal anesthetic care for these patients, leading to decreased complications and contributing to best possible outcomes, will have great value. This article reviews the anesthetic considerations for intraoperative care of geriatric patients and focuses on 3 procedures (hip fractures, emergency abdominal surgery, and transcatheter aortic valve replacement). An approach to evaluation and management of the elderly surgical patient is described.

Postoperative delirium, a common complication in older surgical patients, is independently associated with increased morbidity and mortality. Patients older than 65 years receive greater than one-third of the more than 40 million anesthetics delivered yearly in the United States. This number is expected to increase with the aging of the population. Thus, it is increasingly important that perioperative clinicians who care for geriatric patients have an understanding of the complex syndrome of postoperative delirium.

Postoperative cognitive dysfunction (POCD) is a common complication associated with significant morbidity and mortality in elderly patients. There is much interest in and controversy about POCD, reflected partly in the increasing number of articles published on POCD recently. Recent work suggests surgery may also be associated with cognitive improvement in some patients, termed postoperative cognitive improvement (POCI). As the number of surgeries performed worldwide approaches 250 million per year, optimizing postoperative cognitive function and preventing/treating POCD are major public health issues. In this article, we review the literature on POCD and POCI, and discuss current research challenges in this area.

Medical care of the geriatric patient is an important area of focus as the population ages and life expectancy increases. In particular, critical care of the geriatric patient will be especially affected, because geriatric patients will consume most critical care beds in the future and subsequently require increased use of resources. This review focuses on the physiologic effects of aging on all body systems. Focus on frailty and its effect on recovery from critical illness and its potential to modify the course of patient care will be important areas of research in the future.

> Adequate treatment of pain is of utmost importance in making uncompli-cated the perioperative course for geriatric surgical patients. Effective analgesia reduces morbidity, improves patient and family satisfaction, and is a natural expectation of high-quality care. Pain treatment in older adults is more complicated than in younger counterparts, and great consideration must be given to age-related changes in physiology and pharmacokinetics. Pain treatment must be individualized based on each patient's profile. Side effects must be minimized and organ toxicity avoided. When complications occur they may be more severe, and treat-ment must be prompt. Alternative plans for analgesia must be readily enacted.

> This review summarizes existing evidence relevant to the epidemiology of chronic pain in older adults, age-related differences relevant to pain, pain assessment, and important considerations regarding pain management in later life. Features unique to pain assessment in older adults include the likelihood of multiple diagnoses contributing to chronic pain, the ability of older adults to self-report, including those with mild to moderate cogni-tive impairment, and recognition that some older adults with cognitive impairment may demonstrate various behaviors to communicate pain. Management is best accomplished through a multimodal approach, including pharmacologic and nonpharmacologic treatments, physical rehabilitation, and psychological therapies. Interventional pain therapies may be appropriate in select older adults, which may reduce the need for pharmacologic treatments.

> Many seriously ill geriatric patients are at higher risk for perioperative morbidity and mortality, and incorporating proactive palliative care princi-ples may be appropriate. Advanced care planning is a hallmark of palliative care in that it facilitates alignment of the goals of care between the patient and the health care team. When these goals conflict, perioperative dilemmas can occur. Anesthesiologists must overcome many cultural and religious barriers when managing the care of these patients. Palliative care is gaining ground in several perioperative populations where inte-gration with certain patient groups has occurred. Geriatric anesthesiolo-gists must be aware of how palliative care and hospice influence and enhance the care of elderly patients.

ANESTHESIOLOGY CLINICS

THE CLINICS ARE AVAILABLE ONLINE!
Access your subscription at:
www.theclinics.com

RELATED INTEREST

Foreword

Geriatric Anesthesia: Can We Achieve the Goal of Returning our Elderly to Baseline or Improved Function?

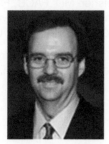

Lee A. Fleisher, MD, FACC, FAHA
Consulting Editor

The importance of age on mortality has been known for decades. It is well known that comorbidities increase with age, but there is great variability between adults of the same age. We all know of the frail elderly who requires all of our talents to "get them through the operation" as opposed to the healthy individual who is still playing three sets of tennis. Yet, recent research has clearly demonstrated that there is significant organ dysfunction postoperatively, including postoperative cognitive changes in this group. In addition, recent research incorporating postdischarge (30-day and 1-year) mortality has demonstrated that the actual rate of death is much higher than was traditionally thought. It is for this reason that the current issue of *Anesthesiology Clinics* was commissioned. It includes a diverse group of articles that span the entire perioperative period and includes chronic pain issues. It also includes a surgeon's perspective since care of the elderly is clearly a team sport. Finally, we should recognize that surgery may not always be the optimal patient-oriented care plan, and palliation should be considered. Therefore, this issue should serve as a resource for all of us who provide care for the elderly.

In order to create such an issue, I was able to enlist two outstanding young investigators to be the coeditors. Mark Neuman, MD, MSc trained in anesthesiology and completed the Robert Wood Johnson Clinical Scholars Program. He is currently Assistant Professor of Anesthesiology and Critical Care at the Perelman School of Medicine at the University of Pennsylvania with joint appointments as an Assistant Professor of Medicine (Geriatrics) and Senior Fellow in Penn's Leonard Davis Institute of Health Economics. He has recently been awarded a major, multicenter pragmatic trial of

Anesthesiology Clin 33 (2015) xiii–xiv
http://dx.doi.org/10.1016/j.anclin.2015.06.002
1932-2275/15/$ – see front matter © 2015 Published by Elsevier Inc.

spinal versus general anesthesia from the Patient Centered Outcomes Research Institute and is the 2015 ASA Presidential Scholar. Charles Brown, MD completed residencies in both anesthesiology and emergency medicine. He is Assistant Professor of Anesthesiology and Critical Care Medicine at the Johns Hopkins School of Medicine. He received a Research Career Development Core Award from the NIH-funded Johns Hopkins Claude D. Pepper Older Americans Independence Center. His research interests include quality and outcomes regarding perioperative management of older adults, specifically focused on postoperative delirium, cognitive change, and transfusion practices.

Lee A. Fleisher, MD, FACC, FAHA
Perelman School of Medicine at the University of Pennsylvania
Philadelphia, PA 19104, USA

E-mail address:
Lee.fleisher@uphs.upenn.edu

Preface

Optimizing Perioperative Care for Older Adults

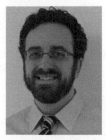 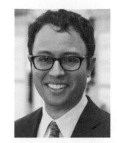

Charles H. Brown IV, MD, MHS   Mark D. Neuman, MD, MSc
Editors

There is a growing wave of older adults presenting for surgery in the United States, and the numbers of the "oldest old" are increasing in parallel. Taking care of a 90-year-old for cardiac surgery is now routine. Although some older adults are robust, the resilience of many older adults has decreased dramatically, and the consequences of any perioperative complications are more profound. Thus, the care of older adults represents an area where excellent anesthetic care can have outsized consequences for a patient's successful recovery.

This issue of *Anesthesiology Clinics* is devoted to the perioperative management of older adults. Importantly, since no specialty can improve outcomes for older adults after surgery in isolation, we have sought the perspective of multiple specialists, including surgeons, anesthesiologists, intensivists, and pain physicians to contribute to this issue. With a diverse selection of articles, we examine the entire spectrum of perioperative care for older adults.

In the preoperative period, we describe new perspectives on optimal preoperative assessment for geriatric patients and highlight a surgical practice that has incorporated these principles into routine practice. Intraoperatively, we describe important physiologic and pharmacologic considerations that are foundations for management of older adults as well as principles of anesthetic care for surgeries that are common in older adults, including transcatheter aortic valve replacement. Finally, in the postoperative period, we present important considerations for older adults needing critical care admission, acute and chronic pain management, and palliative care.

Importantly, neurocognitive changes after surgery are of particular concern in the geriatric patient, and in this issue, we highlight the problems of delirium and postoperative cognitive decline in older adults. We present current knowledge on epidemiology, pathophysiology, risk-stratification, and strategies to prevent these complications.

Anesthesiology Clin 33 (2015) xv–xvi
http://dx.doi.org/10.1016/j.anclin.2015.06.001   **anesthesiology.theclinics.com**
1932-2275/15/$ – see front matter © 2015 Published by Elsevier Inc.

There is both tremendous opportunity and tremendous need to improve the perioperative care of older adults. We are honored to present important topics in geriatric anesthesia in this issue, with the hope that research efforts focused on older adults and collaborations among specialties in the perioperative arena will lead to improving outcomes in the growing number of older adults undergoing surgery.

Charles H. Brown IV, MD, MHS
Division of Cardiac Anesthesia
Department of Anesthesiology
and Critical Care Medicine
Johns Hopkins School of Medicine
Zayed 6208
1800 Orleans Street
Baltimore, MD 21287, USA

Mark D. Neuman, MD, MSc
Department of Anesthesiology
and Critical Care
Perelman School of Medicine
at the University of Pennsylvania
308 Blockley Hall
423 Guardian Drive
Philadelphia, PA 19104, USA

E-mail addresses:
cbrownv@jhmi.edu (C.H. Brown)
neumanm@mail.med.upenn.edu (M.D. Neuman)

The History of Geriatric Anesthesia in the United States and the Society for the Advancement of Geriatric Anesthesia

G. Alec Rooke, MD, PhD

KEYWORDS

- Geriatric • Anesthesiology • Aging • Elderly • Aging population • History

KEY POINTS

- Interest in older patients within the specialty of anesthesiology has existed for at least 60 years.
- The American Society of Anesthesiologists Committee on Geriatric Anesthesia and the Society for the Advancement of Geriatric Anesthesia have been responsible for most educational material available on geriatric anesthesia.
- The American Geriatrics Society has played a major role in raising the profile of aging in the specialty of anesthesiology and in many surgical specialties.
- There are only a modest number of anesthesiologists whose research and academic focus is on the aging patient.

INTRODUCTION

Geriatric anesthesia as focus of interest is a rare phenomenon, even in the current climate of increasing numbers of older patients having surgery. Sixty years ago only a handful of anesthesiologists likely had such a focus. Although the numbers of anesthesiologists whose educational and/or research interests emphasize geriatric anesthesia is still small, the infrastructure to encourage and support such individuals has progressed immeasurably. This article describes how this subspecialty developed and what has been accomplished in the past 60 years. Much of the progress has come from the efforts of the American Society of Anesthesiologists (ASA) Committee on Geriatric Anesthesia, outreach programs by the American Geriatrics Society (AGS), and the Society for the Advancement of Geriatric Anesthesia (SAGA).

The author has no disclosures.
Department of Anesthesiology and Pain Medicine, University of Washington, Box 356540, 1959 Northeast Pacific Street, Seattle, WA 98195-6540, USA
E-mail address: rooke@uw.edu

Anesthesiology Clin 33 (2015) 427–437
http://dx.doi.org/10.1016/j.anclin.2015.05.001
1932-2275/15/$ – see front matter © 2015 Elsevier Inc. All rights reserved.
anesthesiology.theclinics.com

THE EARLY YEARS

Interest in geriatrics within the specialty of anesthesiology has been present for seven decades, with a review article on geriatric anesthesia by Emery Rovenstine published in the very first edition of the journal *Geriatrics*, and perhaps the first textbook on the topic having been published in 1955.[1,2] What is particularly interesting about the textbook is that there are only 39 references, and none of the citations that involve aging came from the anesthesia literature. The same book author then published another text in 1964,[3] but thereafter a full 20 years passed before more books or monographs were published in the 1980s.[4–8] Despite the apparent interest in the field as illustrated by these texts, there was very little available in the way of continuing medical education on geriatric anesthesia. In the 1980s Drs Charles McLeskey and Stanley Muravchick provided refresher course style lectures on geriatric anesthesia at major anesthesia meetings and the occasional state society meeting, but that was about it (Charles McLeskey and Stanley Muravchick, personal communication, 2015). Only one panel on geriatric anesthesia at a major meeting comes to mind, in 1985, organized by Dr McLeskey.

The one exception to this general lack of continuing medical education was the annual Geriatric Anesthesia Symposium held at Washington University beginning in 1974. Dr C. Ronald Stephen, who was then chair of the Department of Anesthesiology, considered geriatric anesthesia an underappreciated field, not only clinically but also with respect to research. He recognized that older patients did not respond the same way to anesthesia as did younger patients, and hoped that an annual symposium would stimulate research on the topic (William Owens, personal communication, 2015). Dr Stephen picked Veterans Day weekend because the ASA calendar was always empty. Dr William Owens was placed in charge of meeting organization and educational program, a position he largely continued even after he became chair at Washington University. This symposium remains the only successful stand-alone annual meeting on geriatric anesthesia ever in the United States, and over the years featured many speakers who would later become prominent in the field. Eventually attendance began to wane, perhaps in part because educational offerings in geriatric anesthesia became more common at other, larger meetings, and the last symposium was held in 1994.

AMERICAN SOCIETY OF ANESTHESIOLOGISTS COMMITTEE ON GERIATRIC ANESTHESIA

The field began to gather momentum in the early 1990s when the ASA initiated their Committee on Geriatric Anesthesia in 1992. The initial chair, Dr Susan Krechel, was a former member of the Department of Anesthesiology at Washington University in St. Louis. Perhaps the highlight of her 4 years as chair was organizing the ASA Workshop on the Care of the Geriatric Patient: Anesthesia and Public Relations, held in San Diego in February, 1995. The program was excellent, but attendance was sparse. A portion of the program was repeated as a symposium at the ASA Annual Meeting that fall, with reasonable attendance. Thereafter the Committee focused on providing panels for the ASA annual meeting and has contributed to the development of at least one panel for all but one ASA annual meeting from 1998 onward. Four more textbooks on geriatric anesthesia were published in the 1990s.[9–12]

During his year as Committee Chair in 1996, Dr J. G. Reves organized the Consensus Conference on Surgery and the Elderly that was held in Durham, North Carolina in September 1997. This meeting brought together anesthesiologists, surgeons, gerontologists, and representatives from the AGS and the National Institutes of Health to identify gaps in knowledge of how age confers perioperative risk and to identify areas of research that would improve understanding of the mechanisms of injury and organ protection in the elderly. A similar meeting was held in 2001. The major topic of discussion was the neurologic effects of anesthesia, and the concern that postoperative delirium and postoperative cognitive change were often considered synonymous in the literature.

A major focus of the Committee has been to promote education on geriatric anesthesia. The initial aim was to improve resident education. In 1998, Dr Rooke distributed a survey to all anesthesiology residency programs with 52 of 144 responses. Most programs described modest formal lectures (2–3 hours), although nine admitted to having no lectures at all. Considerable interest was expressed in a proposed syllabus on geriatric anesthesiology, and some programs that responded to the survey provided volunteers to help write it. This monograph of short articles was designed to be quick reading and useful to private practitioners and the teaching of anesthesia residents. The ASA accepted the syllabus as a work project and made it available on the ASA Web site for many years, and it is still available on the SAGA Web site.[13]

The Committee then turned to educational products geared more to anesthesiologists in active practice. Under the leadership of then Committee chair (and SAGA President) Sheila Barnett, two more work products were organized: the Geriatric Curriculum, completed in 2007; and the Frequently Asked Questions, completed in 2009.[14,15] The Curriculum is a series of topics with a short list of goals; objectives; and most importantly, short lists of key reference articles. The Frequently Asked Questions is a series of questions that are then answered in one or two paragraphs. Not surprisingly, most of the documents were written by Committee and/or SAGA members. The Committee has also been involved in the 2000 and 2005 updates to the ASA patient pamphlet entitled, "Anesthesia for the Senior Citizen."

The Committee also recognized that resident education could be stimulated by making geriatric anesthesia more prominent in the content outline for, and questions in, the American Board of Anesthesiology/ASA Joint Council In-Training Examination. This interest was initiated by Dr Krechel who wrote and encouraged others, myself included, to construct questions for the examinations. SAGA member Dr Raymond Roy was on that council from 1993 to 2005 and Chair from 1998 to 2002. Initially, the only appearance of the terms "geriatric" or "aging" was in the premedications topic, a sub-sub-sub-sub category in the Clinical Sciences section of the Content Outline. He worked hard to increase the appearance of geriatric topics on the content outline for the examination. Resistance was significant, however, because of a prevailing attitude that most issues pertinent to geriatrics were covered, at least indirectly, by topics that related to chronic disease states or drug administration. In 2003, the Joint Council did add "Geriatrics" under the Clinical Subspecialties heading of the content outline. Within the "Geriatrics" category, pharmacologic and physiologic changes were added as specific subheadings. Dr Roy (personal communication, 2015) reports that the creation of SAGA helped promote the subspecialty, as did numerous textbooks published during those years. In consequence, the Joint Council eventually recognized that aging was a process separate from chronic disease, which led to the Content Outline additions.

SOCIETY FOR THE ADVANCEMENT OF GERIATRIC ANESTHESIA

At the time the syllabus was created, it became apparent that there was more interest in geriatric anesthesia within the ranks of the ASA than ever before. Many of the article authors for the syllabus were not committee members, and far more people were expressing interest in the committee than could possibly be accommodated by the committee. The desire to provide a venue for those interested in geriatric anesthesia became the initial driving force for the creation of SAGA. A group of 20 interested persons met during the ASA meeting in October 2000. Proposed bylaws had been prepared in advance by Dr Alec Rooke with more than considerable help and superb advice from Gary Hoorman, an ASA employee. Besides voting to create a society, details of its structure were discussed. The thorniest question revolved around who the new society was to represent. Many believed that nonanesthesiologists and nonphysicians should be full members of the society, whereas others did not want to risk the society potentially losing its focus on the anesthesiologist's perspective. Although not decided at that meeting, it was eventually agreed that only physician or doctoral members would be allowed to vote and hold office. The last item of business was election of officers with Alec Rooke elected President; Jeff Silverstein, President-Elect; Terri Monk, Secretary; and Sheila Barnett, Treasurer.

During the following year, the officers worked out the details of the Bylaws and the name of the society, and the Treasurer began collecting dues. Alec Rooke completed the paperwork to get SAGA established as a nonprofit corporation in the State of Washington in June 2001, and filed the paperwork with the Internal Revenue Service to establish SAGA as a 501(c) (3) charitable organization. At the SAGA meeting held in October 2001 in New Orleans, an attendance of 28 approved the Bylaws and elected the first three at-large Board members. In 2002, the SAGA Web site (www.sagahq.org) was created, in large part because of the volunteer efforts of anesthesiologist Dr Michael Smith and that of his company, Sarker Web Design. In 2005 the Internal Revenue Service issued a final ruling that confirmed SAGA as charitable organization.

The efforts of the ASA Committee on Geriatric Anesthesia and SAGA quickly became deeply intertwined. This relationship is not surprising because SAGA grew out of the limitations to Committee membership. From 2001 on, more than 80% of the Committee members have been SAGA members at one time or another. The level of interaction between SAGA and the Committee is further illustrated in **Table 1**, which shows the relationship of just the SAGA officers to the Committee over the years. There is major benefit to the relationship beyond that both groups have similar interests and goals. When the Committee has an extensive project, or needs speakers for geriatric programs at the ASA meeting, it can tap the membership of SAGA. SAGA is a small society, whereas the ASA carries more clout. When our specialty needs representation with outside organizations, the ASA turns to Committee members, but they are likely to be SAGA members as well. Nevertheless, there are some things that are easier for SAGA to accomplish than having to get ASA leadership approval, and the larger and more stable membership base of SAGA compared with the Committee permits more long-term activities.

Given the minimal success of the ASA workshop and the demise of the Geriatric Anesthesia Symposium mentioned previously, SAGA decided that the best strategy would be to provide educational programs at meetings of other, established societies (**Table 2**). Over the years SAGA has been fortunate to find such interest from several large societies, most notably the Society for Ambulatory Anesthesia and the Society of Cardiovascular Anesthesiologists in addition to the ASA. SAGA has been involved with several small meetings in which it was a cosponsor with respect to the program development. This includes an association, largely driven by Dr Jacques Chelly, with the Orthopedic Anesthesia Pain and Rehabilitation Society that held an annual meeting the day before the start of the ASA annual meeting. From 2009 through 2013, approximately half of the talks at the meeting were oriented toward aging. Eventually the difficulty of having a Friday meeting before the start of the ASA annual meeting got to be too much and the meeting ended in 2013. During this time SAGA and the Orthopedic

Table 1
SAGA officers and their involvement in the ASA Committee of Geriatric Anesthesia

Individual	SAGA Involvement	Committee Involvement
Alec Rooke	President 2001, 2002	Chair 1997, 1998, 2000, 2001, 2005, 2006; Member, 16 y
Jeff Silverstein	President 2003, 2004	Chair 2002, 2003, 2004; Member, 18 y
Terri Monk	President 2005, 2006	Member, 13 y
Sheila Barnett	President 2007, 2008	Chair 2007, 2008, 2009, 2010; Member, 12 y
Chris Jankowski	President 2009, 2010	Member, 5 y
Frederick Sieber	President 2011, 2012	Member, 8 y
Zhongcong Xie	President 2013, 2014	Member, 9 y
Michael Lewis	President 2015, 2016	Chair 2011, 2012; Member, 9 y
Timothy Gilbert	Secretary 2005, 2006	—
Jerome O'Hara	Treasurer 2005, 2006	—
Deborah Culley	Treasurer 2007, 2008	Member, 12 y
Mark Neuman	Secretary 2011, 2012, 2015, 2016	Chair 2015; Member, 4 y
Shamsuddin Akhtar	Secretary 2013, 2014	Member, 7 y
Ruben Azocar	President-Elect 2015–2016	Chair 2013, 2014; Member, 2 y

For SAGA involvement, only the highest officer position is listed. Many have served SAGA in multiple officer roles. All SAGA officers are listed. For ASA Committee involvement, the years as Chair are listed, and the additional number of years spent as a committee member is noted (through 2015). Every Committee chair as of 1996 has been a member of SAGA (1999 Chair was Ruth Burstrom, SAGA member).

Table 2
SAGA member involvement with panels on geriatric anesthesia

Organization	Years	SAGA Involvement
NYPGA	2001	Moderator, 2 of 4 speakers
SAMBA Annual Meeting	2002, 2003, 2004, 2012	3 of 3 moderators, 5 of 9 panel speakers, 1 forum participant and 2 speakers
SCA Annual Meeting	Every year from 2003 through 2012	10 of 10 moderators, 15 of 30 speakers
OAPRS/SAGA pre-ASA meeting	Every year from 2009 through 2013	15 speakers
ASA Annual Meeting	One or more panels from 2001–2014, except 2004	22 of 23 moderators, 60 of 85 speakers
AGS Annual Meeting	2000, 2004	4 of 5 speakers
Age Anesthesia Society (Manchester, England)	2007	7 lectures
2nd International Meeting on Geriatric Anesthesia (Hospital for Special Surgery)	2008	Co-Organizer, 5 lectures
Global Conference on Perioperative Medicine (MD Anderson Cancer Center)	2012	Course Organizer, 6 lectures

Abbreviations: NYPGA, New York Post Graduate Assembly in Anesthesiology; OAPRS, Orthopedic Anesthesia Pain and Rehabilitation Society; SAMBA, Society for Ambulatory Anesthesia; SCA, Society of Cardiovascular Anesthesiologists.

Anesthesia Pain and Rehabilitation Society became even more interconnected as membership discounts were offered for joint memberships. In 2012, the anesthesia department at MD Anderson Cancer Center began an annual meeting on cancer care and how it relates to anesthesia. Their inaugural meeting, organized by SAGA member Dr Vijaya Gottumukkala at MD Anderson, not only focused on cancer care, but also anesthesia for the elderly patient.

SAGA has been involved with two meetings solely dedicated to geriatric anesthesia. The first was held in England in 2007 and was sponsored by the Age Anesthesia Association, the UK equivalent of SAGA, and organized by then Age Anesthesia Association President Andrew Severn. This was followed by a similar meeting organized by SAGA, Age Anesthesia Association, and Nigel Sharrock of the Hospital for Special Surgery in New York City where the meeting was held. Both were superb meetings with great discussions and debate, but unfortunately, at least on this side of the Atlantic Ocean, not well attended by people outside of the sponsoring organizations.

SAGA and Committee members have also provided innumerable talks at many other meetings throughout the United States, such as state society meetings or departmental grand rounds. In addition, SAGA members have been editors of five of the seven textbooks on geriatric anesthesia published in the English language since 2000[16–22] and contributed many articles to those texts.

SAGA holds its own annual meeting. These are fun affairs. Light food and drinks are served, and there is a social hour before the start of the meeting to give people a chance to catch up with long distance friends. Besides a business meeting, there are also invited talks not only by SAGA members but also by guest speakers. Postoperative delirium and cognitive dysfunction have been the most frequent topics of scientific presentations, but other topics have included the state-of-the-art of geriatric anesthesia in other countries, the perspective of a journal editor and an industry representative on geriatric anesthesia, and an overview of reimbursement for geriatric care by the government.

SAGA has also been interested in encouraging research. Although its finances are too modest to provide significant funding, the society has donated $2000 annually as of 2007 to the Foundation for Anesthesia Education and Research to support research and educational grants with a geriatric focus. This level of donation is not trivial to SAGA because the amount represents more than one-third of the society's average annual income. Although SAGA is not directly involved in research, its members have been active in producing original research papers, primarily in the fields of postoperative delirium and postoperative cognitive dysfunction. Not surprisingly, these complications have also been frequent topics at SAGA-organized educational programs.

INVOLVEMENT BY THE AMERICAN GERIATRICS SOCIETY

Perhaps the most significant event in the development of geriatric anesthesia was when the AGS became interested in promoting geriatrics in nonmedical specialties. Beginning in 1994 via funding from the Hartford Foundation, the AGS launched the Geriatrics for Specialists Project to increase the interest in geriatrics among a variety of nonmedical specialties.[23] Initially, the involved specialties were emergency medicine, general surgery, gynecology, orthopedic surgery, and urology. In 1997, anesthesiology, ophthalmology, otolaryngology, physical medicine and rehabilitation, and thoracic surgery were added. In the early stages, representatives from the specialties plus selected geriatricians attended advisory meetings sponsored by the AGS to determine what steps should be taken to promote geriatric education and research.

This group, known as the Interdisciplinary Leadership Group (ILG), made recommendations for a variety of projects to be funded by the AGS. The initial grants were modest in amount and were oriented toward improving resident education in geriatrics within the awardee's department. Anesthesiology was represented by grants to the anesthesiology departments at the University of Pennsylvania, the University of Washington, the University of California at San Francisco, and Duke University. The last major contribution of the ILG was a publication that summarized these activities and the rationale for them.[24] Simply put, in addition to the fact that there are far too few geriatricians to provide all necessary care for older patients, care of the elderly touches many specialties and all must understand the differences in approach necessary to provide appropriate care.

Besides promoting education, the AGS wanted to stimulate research. The approach was two-pronged whereby a literature review was conducted and a new, young investigator research award was established. The literature review came to be known as the Research Agenda-Setting Project.[25] This monograph detailed the then state-of-the-art of geriatric knowledge in each of the 10 member specialties, and also made recommendations on where advances need to be made in each field to improve outcomes in older patients. The Anesthesiology section was written by SAGA member David Cook, with an abridged version published separately.[26] Updates were written 3 years later by former SAGA President Chris Jankowski. The research grant was named after Dennis W. Jahnigen, who spearheaded AGS involvement with specialties other than internal medicine until his untimely death 1998.[27] To those of us who had the opportunity to get to know him, even a little, Dr Jahnigen was an inspiring visionary. The Jahnigen Scholars Award was initially supported by the Hartford Foundation and is now supported by a research grant from the National Institutes of Health in the form of the GEMSSTAR award,[28] plus a supplement for professional development from the awardee's specialty (anesthesiologists receive part of this support from Foundation for Anesthesia Education and Research). The award provides the recipient up to $200,000 for a 2-year period. Anesthesiologists have received 10 of these grants out of the 100 awarded in all 10 specialties from 2002 through 2014.

The AGS has incorporated formal involvement of nongeriatricians into their annual meeting. In the late 1990s and early 2000s, meetings with representatives from the surgical specialties and geriatricians occurred on an "as-needed" basis in the form of the loosely organized ILG. This approach changed with the 2001 creation of the Section for Enhancing Geriatric Understanding and Expertise among Surgical and Medical Specialists (SEGUE). SEGUE meets annually at the AGS meeting and has a half-day educational program on perioperative geriatric care in addition to the business meeting of the SEGUE Council. The specialty societies provide financial support for two of their members to attend the SEGUE Council meetings, which plan the future direction of the Geriatrics for Specialists initiatives. In the past, the SEGUE educational program was simultaneous with but separate from the regular AGS meeting. As of 2014, however, the educational component of SEGUE is now fully integrated into the AGS Annual Meeting. For its part, the SEGUE Council was largely responsible for the development of the Jahnigen Scholars Award. Anesthesiology has been an active participant in the SEGUE Council. Jeff Silverstein, former SAGA President, was a member of the Council from 2006 to 2014, and its Chair from 2007 to 2009. SEGUE and the AGS have also continued to promote education. From 2001 to 2009 grants were provided to academic departments to promote educational projects in their specialty that could be shared throughout the specialty.[29] Anesthesiology received nine such grants, and their resultant teaching materials are found in the Geriatrics for Specialists section of the AGS Web site.[30]

Several medical and surgical specialties have produced guideline papers on the care of the older patient in the last few years. Using a literature review and an expert panel that included anesthesiologists, the AGS published a guideline for prevention and management of postoperative delirium.[31] The American Academy of Orthopedic Surgeons recently published a position paper that included a brief summary of spinal versus general anesthesia for repair of hip fractures in elderly patients, the content of which was reviewed by two members of SAGA.[32] With respect to education, the AGS Geriatrics for Specialists Initiative has supported the concept that each specialty should have a set of competences in geriatric patient care that each resident is expected to have by the conclusion of their residency. A position paper defines these competencies for surgical residencies.[33]

AMERICAN SOCIETY OF ANESTHESIOLOGISTS INVOLVEMENT

Within the ASA leadership and the annual meeting, there has been progressive interest in geriatric anesthesia. The ASA very early on recognized the geriatric imperative when the ASA Committee on Geriatric Anesthesia was created more than two decades ago. Both in spirit and financially, the ASA leadership has supported the efforts of the Committee to represent the ASA with other organizations, most notably the AGS. At the ASA meeting, geriatric anesthesia research was included with the Ambulatory Anesthesia subcommittee for inclusion in abstract presentations. More recently, geriatric anesthesia has been approved as an entirely new track that not only will have separate abstract presentations, but will be responsible for determining all the educational programs on geriatric anesthesia at the ASA meeting. This change becomes effective with the 2016 annual meeting. Educational programs on geriatrics have become common at the annual meeting. Besides the panels mentioned previously, there are often several Problem Based Learning Discussions, Clinical Forums, and Refresher Course Lectures on geriatric anesthesia or related topics, such as postoperative delirium and cognitive dysfunction. There have also been some high-profile presentations. In 2003, Dr Terri Monk gave the Rovenstine lecture on "Postoperative Cognitive Dysfunction: The Next Challenge in Geriatric Anesthesia." In 2008, the Foundation for Anesthesia Education and Research dedicated its panel at the ASA annual meeting to the program "Anesthesia and the Elderly Brain: What the Anesthesiologist Needs to Know." The moderator and all four speakers were SAGA members.

FUTURE CONSIDERATIONS

The ASA Committee on Geriatric Anesthesia and SAGA are justifiably proud of its members' accomplishments over the last 25 years. Also gratifying is the increased interest in the field by the general practitioner, at least judging by the very respectable attendance at the geriatric educational programs at the ASA and other societies' annual meetings. Despite these apparent gains, the educational and research activity has come from a relatively small group of individuals. SAGA membership has always been less than 50 dues-paying members and the Committee size has strict limits. Most members are in academic practice and many have had extensive careers in research or education.

So why has SAGA not grown in numbers? There are likely many reasons. Although the average private practice clinician who cares for adults recognizes the increasing importance of this country's aging population, there is somewhat of the attitude that they deal with older patients all the time so why do they need to pay special attention to that demographic? Such statement should not be viewed as cynical; there is some truth to such an attitude. For example, one does not have to be identified as an "expert" in regional anesthesia to use regional techniques in one's practice. Furthermore, and perhaps more importantly, beyond a few basic principles, current knowledge of the physiology of aging and perioperative outcomes does not provide many clear recommendations on how to manage the older patient so as to minimize adverse outcomes. Until clinicians learn more about how their choices for anesthetic management affect patient recovery and complications, there will be no true imperative to learn about geriatric anesthesia. Both arguments can be used to delineate why there might be resistance to geriatric anesthesia becoming a separate subspecialty, at least in the immediate future. Furthermore, and this is my personal opinion, for most practitioners geriatric anesthesia is of interest enough to want some knowledge on the topic but not so interesting as to really want to be known as someone who specializes in older patients.

There may also be a financial aspect to not wanting to specialize in geriatric anesthesia. An argument can be made that the rapid growth of the Society of Cardiovascular Anesthesiologists was in part stimulated by the higher reimbursement for cardiac anesthesia than for other types of cases, and therefore the anesthesiologists providing such care wanted to be identified as being special. In contrast, SAGA is asking practitioners to take a special interest in caring for a population that is not only challenging and often high risk, but will result in diminished reimbursement, thanks to the backward thinking of the federal government.[34]

SAGA will continue to exist, even thrive perhaps, in the current environment. But until there is a "hook" that provides more than intellectual interest, it seems doubtful that SAGA will ever have a large membership. The impetus is coming, however, with the growing recognition of the impending demographic crises in this country, as noted by the Institutes of Medicine.[35] What will finally provide the key to spark general interest in geriatric anesthesia? On this question the author's crystal ball is a little hazy. Certainly higher reimbursement would help, especially if tied to demonstration of greater expertise in the field or improved patient outcome. The only part of the equation that is clear, however, is that the members of SAGA and the ASA Committee on Geriatric Anesthesia will be there to help the specialty meet the challenge of caring for the older patient.

REFERENCES

1. Rovenstine EA. Geriatric anesthesia. Geriatrics 1946;1:46–53.
2. Lorhan PH. Geriatric anesthesia. Springfield (IL): Charles C. Thomas; 1955.
3. Lorhan PH. International anesthesiology clinics: geriatric anesthesia. Boston: Little, Brown; 1964.
4. Krechel SW. Anesthesia and the geriatric patient. Orlando (FL): Grune & Stratton, Inc; 1984.
5. Stephen CR. Geriatric anesthesia: principles and practice. Oxford (United Kingdom): Butterworth-Heinemann Ltd; 1986.
6. Felts JA. Anesthesia and the geriatric patient. Philadelphia: W. B. Saunders; 1986.
7. Davenport HT. Anaesthesia in the elderly. Oxford (United Kingdom): Butterworth-Heinemann Ltd; 1986.
8. Davenport HT. Anaesthesia and the aged patient. Oxford (United Kingdom): Blackwell Science Ltd; 1988.
9. Gurkowski MA, Smith RB. Anesthesia and pain control in the geriatric patient. Arlington (TX): McGraw-Hill; 1995.
10. McLeskey CH. Geriatric anesthesiology. 1st edition. Baltimore (MD): Williams & Wilkins; 1997.

11. Muravchick S. Geroanesthesia: principles for management of the elderly patient. St Louis (MO): Mosby-Year Book, Inc; 1997.
12. Dauchot PF, Cascorbi H. Problems in anesthesia: management of the elderly surgical patient. Philadelphia: Lippincott-Raven; 1997.
13. American Society of Anesthesiologists Committee on Geriatric Anesthesiology. Syllabus on geriatric anesthesia. 2002. Available at: http://sagahq.org/images/Syllabus.pdf. Accessed June 3, 2015.
14. American Society of Anesthesiologists Committee on Geriatric Anesthesia and the Society for the Advancement of Geriatric Anesthesiology. A geriatric anesthesiology curriculum. 2007. Available at: http://www.asahq.org/resources/clinical-information/geriatric-curriculum   or   http://sagahq.org/images/GeriCurric.pdf. Accessed June 3, 2015.
15. American Society of Anesthesiologists Committee on Geriatric Anesthesia and the Society for the Advancement of Geriatric Anesthesiology. Frequently asked questions about anesthetic considerations for elderly patients. 2009. Available at: http://ecommerce.asahq.org/publicationsAndServices/FAQsAbout AnestheticConsiderationsforElderlyPatients.pdf   or   http://sagahq.org/images/FAQs.pdf. Accessed June 3, 2015.
16. Silverstein JH. Anesthesiology Clinics of North America: geriatric anesthesia. Philadelphia: WB Saunders Co; 2000. Available at: http://sagahq.org/images/GeriCurric.pdf.
17. Sieber F. Geriatric anesthesia. New York: McGraw-Hill Professional; 2006.
18. Silverstein JH, Rooke GA, Reves JG, et al. Geriatric anesthesiology. 2nd edition. New York: Springer Science+Business Media; 2008.
19. Kumra VP. Applied geriatric anesthesia. London: Jaypee Brothers Medical Pub; 2009.
20. Silverstein JH. Anesthesiology clinics: problems with geriatric anesthesia patients. St Louis (MO): W. B. Saunders; 2009.
21. Barnett SR. Manual of geriatric anesthesia. New York: Springer; 2013.
22. Dodds C, Kumar C. Oxford textbook of anaesthesia for the elderly patient. New York: Oxford University Press; 2014.
23. Solomon DH, Burton JR, Lundebjerg NE, et al. The new frontier: increasing geriatrics expertise in surgical and medical specialties. J Am Geriatr Soc 2000;48:702-4.
24. Solomon DH. A statement of principles: toward improved care of older patients in surgical and medical specialties. The interdisciplinary leadership group of the American Geriatrics Society project to increase geriatrics expertise in surgical and medical specialties. J Am Geriatr Soc 2000;48(6):699-701.
25. Available at: http://newfrontiers.americangeriatrics.org/. Accessed June 3, 2015.
26. Cook DJ, Rooke GA. Priorities in perioperative geriatrics. Anesth Analg 2003;96:1823-36.
27. Katz PR, Burton JR, Drach GW, et al. The Jahnigen scholars program: a model for faculty career development. J Am Geriatr Soc 2009;57:2324-7.
28. Available   at: http://www.nia.nih.gov/research/dgcg/grants-early-medical-surgical-specialists-transition-aging-research-gemsstar. Accessed June 3, 2015.
29. Potter JF, Burton JR, Drach GW, et al. Geriatrics for residents in the surgical and medical specialties: implementation of curricula and training experiences. J Am Geriatr Soc 2005;53:511-5.
30. Available   at: http://www.americangeriatrics.org/gsi/who_is_gsi/gsi_mission_goals. Accessed June 3, 2015.

31. The American Geriatrics Society Expert Panel on Postoperative Delirium in Older Adults. Postoperative delirium in older adults: best practice statement from the American Geriatrics Society. J Am Coll Surg 2015;220(2):136–48.
32. American Academy of Orthopaedic Surgeons. Management of hip fractures in the elderly: evidence-based clinical practice guideline. 2014. Available at: http://www.aaos.org/research/guidelines/HipFxGuideline_rev.pdf. Accessed June 3, 2015.
33. Bell RH, Drach GW, Rosenthal RA. Proposed competencies in geriatric patient care for use in assessment for initial and continued board certification of surgical specialists. J Am Coll Surg 2011;213(5):683–90.
34. Rooke GA. Anesthesia for the older patient. In: Barash P, Cullen B, Stoelting R, et al, editors. Clinical anesthesia. 7th edition. Philadelphia: Lippincott Williams & Wilkins; 2013. p. 891–904.
35. Retooling for an aging America: building the health care workforce. Available at: http://www.nap.edu/catalog/12089.html. Accessed June 3, 2015.

Geriatrics and the Perioperative Surgical Home

Matthew T. Mello, MD[a],*, Ruben J. Azocar, MD[b],
Michael C. Lewis, MBBS[c]

KEYWORDS

- Perioperative surgical home • Enhanced recovery after surgery • Triple aim
- Integrator/perioperative physician • Geriatric surgical home

KEY POINTS

- Select patients/procedures will be the initial construct of the perioperative surgical home to be effective. This is noted by the success seen at University of California Irvine Medical Center Joint Replacement Surgical Home.
- By 2030, the US population older than 65 years is expected to be 19%; therefore, this larger geriatric population will be presenting for elective surgery, and with their age-related comorbidities are at increased risk for perioperative complications.
- With the development of necessary health care reform along with the aging patient population, the American Society of Anesthesiologists (ASA) has introduced the concept of the perioperative surgical home in which the anesthesiologist serves as leader or integrator of the patient's care team throughout the perioperative period to improve patient outcomes, enhancing the quality of care and reducing health care costs.

INTRODUCTION

The perioperative surgical home (PSH) is a physician-led, patient-centered, interdisciplinary, and team-based system of coordinated patient care. Health care in the United States has been under increasing scrutiny due to the accumulation of rising health care costs and the disparaging fragmented quality in its delivery. In order to improve this current fragmented, cost-inefficient system, the PSH may be a push in the right direction. All stakeholders in the delivery of surgical services, as well as the patients themselves, may gain significantly from its successful implementation.

Disclosure: The authors have no relevant financial or nonfinancial disclosures.
[a] University of Florida College of Medicine–Jacksonville, 350 West 7th Street, Jacksonville, FL 32206, USA; [b] Tufts University School of Medicine, Boston, MA, USA; [c] University of Florida College of Medicine–Jacksonville, Jacksonville, FL, USA
* Corresponding author.
E-mail address: matthew.mello@jax.ufl.edu

DEFINITION OF THE PERIOPERATIVE SURGICAL HOME

The evolution of the PSH model is firmly rooted in the triple aim philosophy in that it strives to improve the quality of care, reduce the overall health care expense, and improve the overall health of the population. It represents a potential paradigm of practice in that it contains a patient-centered, physician-led, team-based coordination of care (**Fig. 1**).

If one takes a long-term view of the development of health care in the United States, one sees rapid and significant changes in recent times. Concepts such as patient-centered care and shared decision making represent significant paradigm shifts from the time held current physician-centered care model. A patient-centered model considers the preferences of the patient in making health care decisions; this model has been associated with decreased use of expensive tests and procedures, improved outcomes, and most importantly decreased discomfort and improved patient satisfaction.[1]

Although the PSH is a newer model with limited established supporting data, it would not be unreasonable to extrapolate from the data and literature on enhanced recovery after surgery (ERAS) and practice model outcomes from pioneer institutions in the PSH like University of California Irvine Health as well as other institutions.[2]

The perioperative clinical protocol implemented by ERAS has standardized management of several facets of the perioperative management of patients (**Table 1**).[3–5] This model has shown positive results in reduced length of stay, reduced risk of hospital-acquired infections, improved patient satisfaction, and postoperative outcomes.[6] The PSH model would further incorporate the ideals in ERAS within an extended framework to include coordination of care through a perioperative physician managing the entirety of the perioperative care (**Fig. 2**). Within this paradigm, the perioperative physician allows for much needed continuity of care while creating a care that can evolve within the local environment and make adjustments to strict predefined items.

Within the PSH, the perioperative physician functions to reduce variability of care and stray away from the current fragmented care of several physicians over the patient's perioperative course. The creation of a perioperative continuum, rather than discrete preoperative, intraoperative, postoperative, and postdischarge encounters creates a unique opportunity to gain ground in a failing health care environment by improving outcomes, reducing costs, and improving patient satisfaction.[5] The current fragmented care model creates this nature of running unnecessary tests on patients, due to lack of access or these previously run preoperative diagnostics being lost in a fragmented

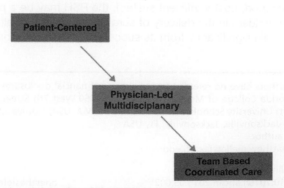

Fig. 1. The triple aim philosophy of the perioperative surgical home model.

Table 1
Common implemented protocols

Preoperative	Intraoperative	Postoperative
Patient counseling	Monitoring	Exercise therapy
Fluid administration guidelines	Body temperature control	Use of nonsteroidal anti-inflammatory drugs with no oral opioids
No fasting; carbohydrate loading	Thoracic epidural	Early mobilization
Minimum bowel preparation	Goal-directed fluid therapy	Stimulation of intestinal motility and early oral intake
No premedication with benzodiazepines	Short-acting anesthetic drugs	Early postoperative resuscitation guidelines
Nutritional goals	PONV prevention	—

Data from Melnyk M, Casey RG, Black P, et al. Enhanced recovery after surgery (ERAS) protocols: time to change practice? Can Urol Assoc J 2011;5(5):342–8.

abyss. Besides the obvious unnecessary running multiples of the same study and increasing health care costs, this also creates dissatisfaction within the patient.

TRIPLE AIM

Political and economic realities have led to widespread pressures to reform the health care delivery system. Any potential change has to recognize and balance the inherent expansion of services in a context of cost containment while improving the quality of care provided. The Institute for Healthcare Improvement (IHI) has created the framework of the triple aim (**Fig. 3**), with 3 interdependent goals:

1. Improving the individual experience and quality of care
2. Improving the overall health of the population
3. Reducing the per capita costs of care

To hold these concepts together and for them to run fluidly with one another, an integrator, or entity in charge of making sure these factions intertwine with one another

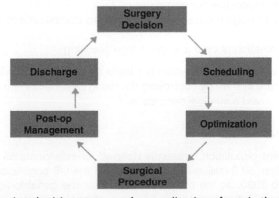

Fig. 2. A perioperative physician manages the coordination of care in the perioperative surgical home model.

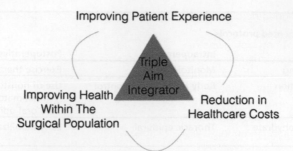

Fig. 3. Triple aim framework created by the Institute for Healthcare Improvement, including 3 interdependent goals.

will typically coordinate the care. This integrator is responsible for achieving the accumulation of the 3 components of the triple aim for a specified population.[7–9]

WHERE TO START?

The transition to a PSH requires selecting the right procedures that have the most to gain. Deciding where to look, one can glimpse into the fastest growing surgical procedures. In 2008, total knee replacement had a cumulative inpatient cost exceeding $9 billion, which offers room for exceptional cost savings if the system can find a way to better the provided health care in a more efficient manner. This avenue proved to be successful for the University of California Irvine Medical Center and its joint replacement surgical home.[10,11]

BENEFITS OF THE PERIOPERATIVE SURGICAL HOME

Proposed benefits of the perioperative surgical home according to the ASA include[12]

1. Reduction in preoperative testing and unnecessary consults
2. Reduction in day of surgery cancellations
3. Improvement in clinical outcomes
4. Development of postprocedural care initiatives: coordination to improve PONV, postoperative pain, and issues with anticoagulation (all to promote better outcomes and shorter length of stay)
5. Reduction in postoperative complications
6. Cost reduction (through reduced testing, reduced complications, and decreased length of stay)
7. Improved coordination of care and discharge planning

These benefits will fuel success within the triple aim model to alleviate the scrutiny on the US health care system by controlling the rising costs and improving the quality of care provided toward a surgical candidate.[12]

AGING PATIENT POPULATION

The geriatric patient population, presently defined as individuals 65 years or older, numbered more than 39.6 million in 2009 (12.9% of the US population) are growing. Moving forward to 2030, as the baby boomers enter the geriatric age group, there will be an estimated 72.1 million people 65 years of age or greater, exceeding twice the number in 2000. This shift in the age curve will place an estimated 19% of the population in this geriatric classification, creating a greater demand on efficient geriatric health care.[13]

The aging population also gives rise to increased prevalence of chronic conditions such as peripheral vascular disease, arthritis, diabetes, cardiac disease, hypertension, and obesity, all of which can complicate the perioperative period, exacerbating morbidity and mortality. Orthopedic surgical procedures have pioneered some of the perioperative surgical home data. If one looks at the geriatric population, one can see osteoporosis incidence coincide and with the increase in age. The prevalence of osteoporosis in people aged 50 years of age or older in the United States is an estimated 10.3%.[14] In a meta-analysis, the 1-year mortality rate following hip fracture in the geriatric US population was 20% in women and 26% in men. Coordinated, multidisciplinary care tailored to patients suffering from hip fractures has been described as protocol-driven and has been shown to be effective.[15–18]

ROLE IN GERIATRICS

The concept of this integrator, or perioperative physician, will allow for a more cohesive health care management in a frail population that typically requires extensive workup for multiple comorbidities.[7–9] In the current model, fragmented care leads to multiple unnecessary tests as part of the workup, with the patient suffering from having multiple plans taking place that do not always coincide. The health care system also feels the financial strain secondary to these unnecessary tests or finds poor timing of the needed test inadequate for quality patient care. By streamlining the system with a perioperative surgical home model, the triple aim of reducing cost, improving quality of care, and improving the overall health of the population can be met through effective protocols and a perioperative physician.

COMPLICATIONS IN THE GERIATRIC POPULATION: ROOM FOR IMPROVEMENT?

The combination of improvements in medicine and better living conditions has led to an increasing proportion of the geriatric population. The increasing elderly population has a coinciding growth in the number of surgical procedures.[19] Outcome studies have demonstrated that the morbidity and mortality numbers in the elderly are substantially increased from their younger counterparts, creating a large need for improved health care in the geriatric population.[20]

Part of the triple aim is to improve surgical outcome. Postoperative complications often dictate surgical outcomes as defined by the quality initiatives measuring the major system-based troubles, neurologic and cardiopulmonary, faced by the geriatric surgical population. Structured protocols as part of the PSH have a positive impact as part of the quality initiatives. In fact, delirium is the most common neurologic complication in the elderly surgical population, with incidence ranging from 15% to 53%, and anesthesia quality initiatives have been implemented as a protocol to be a preventative measure.[19]

The most common complications in the surgical geriatric patient are neurologic, cardiac, and pulmonary.

These complications comprise an incidence of 15%, 12%, and 7%, respectively, more than a third cumulatively. This is a substantial number of patients who could benefit from effective protocols to ease the incidence of these complications.[21]

Fine tuning evidenced-based medicine to create perioperative protocols for common complications like delirium can provide an effective triple aim. Anesthetic choices, early stimulation, and even prophylaxis regimens can prove beneficial to combat postoperative delirium in the elderly population. An example of this is the use of low-dose haloperidol (1.5 mg/d) in vulnerable populations in higher-risk procedures to reduce the severity and length of delirium.[22] Evidenced-based protocols directed by best outcomes can create success within the triple aim framework.

FUTURE CONSIDERATIONS/SUMMARY

Although a newer concept in the infancy stages, the PSH may provide a stepping stone to success in the inevitable changes in health care. This newer idea has limited data of success, but if one can draw on the validated successes of the ERAS program in Europe, or results spawned by the pioneers at the University of Alabama at Birmingham and at University of California Irvine Health, one may have find a credible blueprint for the needed paradigm shift. The success of the PSH has important implications in the surgical care of the geriatric population, as this group of patients has both the most to gain and the most to lose.

Part of the growth of the PSH will be to continue to develop and test best practices for management of elderly patients. Implementation of protocol-driven management will establish an effective surgical home model overseen by a multidisciplinary physician as part of the American Society of Anesthesiologists' Perioperative Surgical Home collaborative.

REFERENCES

1. Adamina M, Kehlet H, Tomlinson GA, et al. Enhanced recovery pathways optimize health outcomes and resource utilization: a meta-analysis of randomized con- trolled trials in colorectal surgery. Surgery 2011;149:830–40.
2. Vetter TR, Goeddel LA, Boudreaux AM, et al. The perioperative surgical home: how can it make the case so everyone wins? BMC Anesthesiol 2013;13:6.
3. Knott A, Pathak S, Mcgrath JS, et al. Consensus views on implementation and measurement of enhanced recovery after surgery in England: Delphi study. BMJ Open 2012;2(6). pii:e001878.
4. Varadhan KK, Neal KR, Dejong CH, et al. The enhanced recovery after surgery (ERAS) pathway for patients undergoing major elective open colorectal surgery: a meta-analysis of randomized controlled trials. Clin Nutr 2010;29(4):434–40.
5. Kain ZN, Vakharia S, Garson L, et al. The perioperative surgical home as a future perioperative practice model. Anesth Analg 2014;118(5):1126–30.
6. Miller TE, Thacker JK, White WD, et al. Reduced length of hospital stay in colorectal surgery after implementation of an enhanced recovery protocol. Anesth Analg 2014;118(5):1052–61.
7. Berwick DM, Nolan TW, Whittington J. The triple aim: care, health, and cost. Health Aff (Millwood) 2008;27(3):759–69.
8. Stiefel M, Nolan K. A guide to measuring the triple aim: population health, experience of care, and per capita cost IHI innovation series white paper. Cambridge (MA): Institute for Healthcare Improvement; 2012.
9. Vetter TR, Boudreaux AM, Jones KA, et al. The perioperative surgical home: how anesthesiology can collaboratively achieve and leverage the triple aim in health care. Anesth Analg 2014;118(5):1131–6.
10. Cisternas MG, Murphy LB, Yelin EH, et al. Trends in medical care expenditures of US adults with arthritis and other rheumatic conditions 1997 to 2005. J Rheumatol 2009;36(11):2531–8.
11. Chaurasia A, Garson L, Kain ZL, et al. Outcomes of a joint replacement surgical home model clinical pathway. Biomed Res Int 2014;2014:296–302.

12. Schweitzer M, Fahy B, Leib M, et al. The perioperative surgical home model. ASA Newsl 2013;77:58–9.
13. U.S. Department of Health & Human Services. Administration of aging. Available at: http://www.aoa.gov/AoARoot/Aging_Statistics. Accessed February 2, 2015.
14. U.S. Census Bureau: an aging world. 2008. Available at: http://www.census.gov/prod/2009pubs/p95-09-1. Accessed February 1, 2015.
15. Haentjens P, Magaziner J, Colón-emeric CS, et al. Meta-analysis: excess mortality after hip fracture among older women and men. Ann Intern Med 2010;152(6):380–90.
16. Management of hip fracture in older people, National Clinical Guideline 111. Scottish Intercollegiate Guidelines Network. 2009. Available at: http://www.sign.ac.uk/pdf/sign111.pdf. Accessed November 12, 2014.
17. Miura LN, Dipiero AR, Homer LD. Effects of a geriatrician-led hip fracture program: improvements in clinical and economic outcomes. J Am Geriatr Soc 2009;57(1):159–67.
18. Watne LO, Torbergsen AC, Conroy S, et al. The effect of a pre- and postoperative orthogeriatric service on cognitive function in patients with hip fracture: randomized controlled trial (Oslo Orthogeriatric Trial). BMC Med 2014;12:63.
19. Sieber FE, Barnett SR. Preventing postoperative complications in the elderly. Anesthesiol Clin 2011;29(1):83–97.
20. Bentrem DJ, Cohen ME, Hynes DM, et al. Identification of specific quality improvement opportunities for the elderly undergoing gastrointestinal surgery. Arch Surg 2009;144(11):1013–20.
21. Liu LL, Leung JM. Predicting adverse postoperative outcomes in patients aged 80 years or older. J Am Geriatr Soc 2000;48(4):405–12.
22. Bourne RS, Tahir TA, Borthwick M, et al. Drug treatment of delirium: past, present and future. J Psychosom Res 2008;65(3):273–82.

Physiology Considerations in Geriatric Patients

Bret D. Alvis, MD, Christopher G. Hughes, MD*

KEYWORDS

- Geriatric • Physiology • Cardiovascular aging • Neurologic aging • Aging

KEY POINTS

- Changes in structure, function, metabolism, and blood flow in the aging brain lead to cognitive impairments, most frequently episodic memory changes, and an increased risk of delirium in the acute setting.
- The geriatric population tends to have higher blood pressure with lower cardiac output and diminished chronotropic and inotropic responses to beta-receptor stimulation.
- Respiratory aging results in changes to mechanical properties of the respiratory system, reduction of arterial oxyhemoglobin saturation, and Impaired response to hypoxia.
- Gastrointestinal changes with aging include altered esophageal motility, delayed gastric emptying, and reduction in hepatic metabolism.
- There is a reduction in renal function with age, and changes also occur to the endocrine system, including diminished tissue responsiveness and reduction in hormone secretion from peripheral glands.

INTRODUCTION

Physiology is a complex, ever-changing state with changes occurring at the structural, functional, and molecular levels as people age.[1] The process of aging is complex and multifactorial with multiple hypotheses broadly categorized into either the programmed theory or the error theory.[1] The programmed theory states that delineated biological alterations in homeostatic state and natural defense occur over time.[1]

Contributions: The authors performed the literature review, prepared the article, and approved the final article.

Disclosure: Dr C.G. Hughes is supported by National Institutes of Health HL111111, R03AG045085 (Bethesda, MD), and Jahnigen Career Development Award sponsored by the American Geriatrics Society (New York, NY).

Conflicts of Interest: None.

Division of Critical Care Medicine, Department of Anesthesiology, Vanderbilt University School of Medicine, 1211 21st Avenue South, 526 MAB, Nashville, TN 37212, USA

* Corresponding author.

E-mail address: christopher.hughes@vanderbilt.edu

The error theory focuses on free radical accumulation secondary to reactive oxygen species generated during mitochondrial energy production, causing oxidative damage to DNA, protein, and lipids.[1] No matter the theory, aging is defined as the normal progressive decline in function and ability to respond to intrinsic (eg, catecholamines, inflammation) or extrinsic (eg, infection, surgery) stimuli.[2]

A patient's age is a strong correlate of risk of morbidity and mortality.[3] For noncardiac surgery, 30-day mortality is expected to increase by a factor of 1.35 per decade of age.[3] Age itself is also an independent risk factor for a long list of diseases, injuries, hospitalization, length of hospitalization, and adverse drug reactions,[4] and almost every organ system is affected by aging. This article therefore discusses the most recent evidence and understanding of how aging affects the major organ systems.

NERVOUS SYSTEM

The aging of the brain is accompanied by a change in structure, function, and metabolism (**Table 1**).[5] The volume and weight of the brain decline at a rate of approximately 5% per decade after age 40 years.[6] Once the brain is 70 years old, the rate of decline is thought to increase.[6] The changes in neuronal volume and affected areas may be related to gender.[6] Brain atrophy starts earlier in men but is more rapid in women once it has started.[5] There are longitudinal studies using MRI and reviews of cross-sectional studies that show the prefrontal cortex as the most affected region of neuronal cell death.[6] The medial temporal lobes are also sensitive to age,[5] and additional areas include the cerebellar vermis, cerebellar hemispheres, and hippocampus.[6]

On analysis of postmortem brains, there is a greater loss of white matter than gray matter with aging,[7] and granular degeneration of myelinated axons is observed regularly by the age of 40 years.[7] Neuronal cell death is thought to be the main reason for the loss of gray matter; however, whether this is the only reason is unclear.[6] There may be additional changes in dendritic arbor, spines, and synapses, with dendritic sprouting occurring to help maintain a similar number of synapses and compensate for any cell death.[6]

Along with a reduction of brain volume, there are cognitive changes associated with aging. Memory declines are one such cognitive change, with decline in episodic memory being most common.[6] This type of memory is defined as "a form of memory in which information is stored with mental tags, about where, when, and how the information was picked up"[6] and is thought to decline starting around the fourth and fifth decades.

Neurotransmitter changes also occur with age. Dopamine levels decline by approximately 10% per decade starting in early adulthood.[6] This decrease has been associated with declines in cognitive and motor performance.[6] Serotonin and brain-derived neurotrophic factor levels also decrease with age, and decreases in these neurotransmitters have been associated with reduced synaptic plasticity regulation and

| Table 1 | | | |
Changes in the neurologic system with age			
Brain volume	▼	Blood-brain barrier permeability	▲
Dopamine levels	▼	Arterial wall thickness	▲
Cerebral metabolic rate	▼	Monoamine oxidase activity	▲

▲, Augmented; ▼, diminished.

neurogenesis.[6] Monoamine oxidase, an important substance in the homeostasis of neurotransmitter levels, increases with age and may liberate free radicals from reactions that exceed inherent antioxidant reserves.[6]

The blood-brain barrier protects the central nervous system from systemic insults through selective permeability. Increasing age is associated with increasing blood-brain barrier permeability,[8] thereby allowing inappropriate passage of mediators from the plasma into the central nervous system. This process likely results in an increased inflammatory response and structural damage in the brain as well as altered patterns of neuronal activity by modulating synthesis of neurotransmitters and changing expression of neurotransmitter receptors.[9,10]

Vascular distribution in the brain also changes every decade of life. Capillaries are densely packed in areas of the brain that have higher processing demands, and these dense areas of capillaries tend to decrease.[7] Starting around the fifth decade of life, every decade shows an increase in the degree and number of microvessel deformities.[7] Cerebroarterial change begins mostly in the intima with approximately 50% of the vessels showing intimal thickening by the fourth decade and up to 80% by the eighth decade.[7] These changes are often the precursors to arteriosclerosis, which increases vascular resistance and decreases perfusion pressure, thereby compromising neurocognitive function.[7] Studies using functional imaging techniques to evaluate the effects of aging have found a reduction in cerebral metabolic rate of oxygen consumption with decreased cerebral blood flow in gray matter but preservation of blood flow to the white matter.[7]

With an aging population, there will be an increase in elderly patients having surgery.[11] With this, the prevalence of postoperative cognitive disorders in the aging brain is likely to increase.[11] All the changes (see **Table 1**) seen in the brain increase the likelihood of postoperative cognitive disorders, including delirium in the acute setting and postoperative cognitive dysfunction in the long term.[11]

CARDIOVASCULAR SYSTEM

The geriatric population tends to have higher blood pressures, similar heart rates and ejection fractions, and lower left ventricular end-diastolic volumes, stroke volumes, and cardiac outputs compared with younger populations (**Table 2**).[3] These aging-related changes in the cardiovascular system primarily start with changes in connective tissues. Connective tissue stiffens within the arteries, veins, and myocardium, causing them to become less compliant.[3] This stiffening is secondary to a

Table 2
Changes in the cardiovascular system with age

Cardiac Changes		Vascular Changes	
Heart weight	▲	Arterial wall thickness	▲
Cardiomyocyte number	▼	Elastin	▼
Collagen cross-linking	▲	Elastin fragmentation	▲
Early diastolic filling	▼	Arterial distensibility	▼
End-diastolic filling	▲	Pulse wave velocity	▲
Chronotropic responsiveness to beta-agonists	▼	Total peripheral resistance	▲
Inotropic responsiveness to beta-agonists	▼	Endothelial function	▼

▲, Augmented; ▼, diminished.

cessation of elastin production in the fourth decade of life.[3] Also, collagen turnover is a slow process, and both elastin and collagen proteins accumulate free radical damage over time.[3] As elastin is damaged, it is then replaced with less flexible collagen protein.[3]

Arterial stiffening leads to systolic hypertension, impaired impedance matching, and myocardial hypertrophy.[3,4] The stiffening within the aorta causes an increase in systolic blood pressure and a decrease in diastolic pressure.[3,4,12] The diminished diastolic pressure leads to a decrease in coronary blood flow.[12] Under normal circumstances, most of the stroke volume is contained within the thoracic aorta; as the aorta stiffens, the pressure to transfer this volume increases.[3] Thus, chronically increased left ventricular afterload leads to left ventricular thickening.[4] There is also an increase in impedance matching between the declining strength of the myocardial contraction and the increases in pressure within the aorta.[3] When this pressure wave travels down the arterial tree, the wave reflects off both the vessel walls and branch points, returning to the thoracic aorta.[3] This pressure reflection creates a poor impedance match and causes more strain on the myocardium, serving as a significant stimulus for myocyte hypertrophy.[3]

The combination of myocyte hypertrophy and increased left ventricular afterload prolongs myocardial contraction.[4] This extended contraction leads to a delay in ventricular relaxation and results in early diastolic filling rates declining by approximately 50% between the second and eighth decades.[4] The end-diastolic volume is typically preserved secondary to late diastolic filling and becomes more reliant on atrial contribution for effective filling.[4] Ventricular myocardial stiffening and hypertrophy, therefore, render the heart dependent on atrial filling pressures.[3] They also increase susceptibility to diastolic heart failure[3] because diastolic dysfunction is a key factor in the development of heart failure with preserved ejection fraction.[13]

Venous stiffening with age decreases ability to buffer changes in blood volume and blood distribution.[3] More than 80% of blood volume is stored within the venous network.[3] This reservoir is therefore important in maintaining a stable preload to the heart, and venous stiffening impairs the ability to keep preload constant.[3]

Aging results in an increase in sympathetic nervous system activity and higher levels of circulating norepinephrine, resulting in an increase in arteriole constriction and systemic vascular resistance.[3] Evidence for this increase in norepinephrine includes an increase in norepinephrine release from nerve terminals, an increase in the percentage of norepinephrine reaching the general circulation, and a decrease in the metabolism and reuptake.[3]

The myocardium's beta-receptor is also affected with age. The response of the receptor to stimulation is reduced, resulting in a decrease in heart rate and contractile response to hypotension, exercise, and catecholamines.[3] This process does not seem to be secondary to a decline in the number of beta-receptors but rather a diminishment in the intracellular coupling with adenylate cyclase.[3] The diminished chronotropic and inotropic response of the heart to beta-receptor stimulation changes the heart's ability to respond to either intrinsic or exogenous catecholamine stimulation.[3] This beta-receptor limitation increases the dependence of the Frank-Starling relationship to maintain cardiac output.[3] Other changes in the cardiovascular system include a diminished baroreflex stimulation, lower vagal nerve tone, and reduced oxygen extraction.[3] The impaired baroreflex system and vagal tone result in less heart rate variability and ability to control a constant cardiac output.[3]

Endothelial dysfunction is a leading theory for the mechanism of vascular aging. Endothelial function, including nitric oxide release, has vasoprotective and cardioprotective properties because of inhibition of platelet aggregation and inflammatory cell adhesion to endothelial cells, disruption of proinflammatory cytokines, apoptosis inhibition, and tissue energy metabolism regulation.[12] There is considerable published evidence showing an increase in reactive oxygen species within the heart and vasculature with age,[14] and the accumulation of oxidative stress results in altered nitric oxide production.[12] Furthermore, there is also a lower production of nitric oxide with age.[12] These factors diminish the bioavailability of nitric oxide in the coronary and peripheral circulation in the elderly, resulting in impairment of flow in the microvasculature and increasing risk for organ dysfunction.[12]

The stiffening of the connective tissue, impaired impedance matching, myocardial hypertrophy, venous stiffening, increase in sympathetic nervous system, altered nitric oxide production, and the diminished beta-receptor response are the changes (see **Table 2**) in the cardiovascular system that cause there to be more hypotension and greater blood pressure lability during anesthesia in elderly patients versus young adults. This alteration affects the depth and type of anesthesia required and the sympathetic nervous system response to changes in surgical stimulus and cardiovascular medications.

RESPIRATORY SYSTEM

The lungs continue to develop throughout life, and maximal functional status is achieved in the early part of the third decade, after which lung function gradually declines.[15] Changes with aging include alteration of the mechanical properties of the respiratory system, reduction of arterial oxyhemoglobin saturation, and impaired response to hypoxia (**Table 3**).[15]

The parenchyma of the lung undergoes significant structural alterations with aging, with the most important change being a reduction in number and crosslinks of elastic fibers resulting in a reduction of elastic recoil.[15-17] This reduction creates inward forces that promote a decrease in lung volumes at an average rate of between 0.1 and 0.2 cm H_2O per year, and this decrease is most pronounced after the fifth decade.[15] Homogeneous enlargement of the air spaces also causes a reduction in alveolar surface area from 75 m^2 to 30 to 60 cm^2 by the age of 70 years, increasing lung compliance and representing functional emphysema.[15,17]

In addition to decreased elastic recoil, there is also a decrease in compliance with age caused by structural changes with intercostal muscles, joints, and rib vertebral articulations that decrease compliance of the chest wall.[15-18] Age-related development of osteoporosis results in a reduction of height of the thoracic vertebrae causing further restriction.[18] In addition, a reduction of respiratory muscle mass may contribute to a decrease in the force produced by the respiratory muscle activity.[15] However, this loss of chest wall muscular function decreases the outward force requirements such that the total lung capacity remains unchanged.[15,18]

Table 3 Changes in the respiratory system with age			
Ventilation-perfusion mismatch	▲	Protective cough	▼
Chest wall rigidity	▲	Residual volume	▲
Respiratory muscle strength	▼	Vital capacity	▼
Work of breathing	▲	Closing volume	▲
Respiratory muscle endurance	▼	Gas exchange	▼
Functional alveolar surface area	▼	Response to hypoxemia and hypercapnia	▼

▲, Augmented; ▼, diminished.

With these changes in the properties of the connective tissues, there are significant changes to the mechanics of the lung. The functional residual capacity increases by 1% to 3% per decade.[15] The residual volume increases by 5% to 10% per decade.[15] Because the total lung capacity remains unchanged, there is a decrease in vital capacity as much as 40% from 20 to 70 years of age.[15] This decrease in physiologic reserve increases geriatric patients' vulnerability to infection and impairment.[16] There are progressive decreases in both forced vital capacity (FVC; 14–30 mL per year) and forced expiratory volume in 1 second (FEV$_1$; 23–32 mL per year).[15] After the age of 65 years, there is a decrease in FEV$_1$ of approximately 38 mL per year.[15] These changes can make a normal FEV$_1$/FVC ratio as low at 55% in the elderly.[15]

Aging also affects gas exchange properties. Arterial oxygenation gradually declines with aging,[15,17] likely secondary to an increase in ventilation/perfusion heterogeneity caused by a decrease in alveolar surface area and the premature closure of small airways.[15,16] To predict the effect of age on arterial oxygenation, several equations have been proposed.[15] Between the ages of 40 and 75 years, the best equation that takes into account both $PaCO_2$ and body mass index (BMI) is Pao_2 (mm Hg) = 143.6 – (0.39 × age) – (0.56 × BMI) – (0.57 × $PaCO_2$).[15] After the age of 75 years, arterial oxygen tension does not correlate with BMI and $PaCO_2$ and instead remains stable at approximately 83 mm Hg.[15]

Elderly people have a lower tidal volume and a higher respiratory rate than younger people.[15] There is an approximately 50% decrease in their response to hypoxia and hypercapnia[15] and a decrease in diffusion capacity of the lung.[16] Increased ventilation is often required to compensate for this decreased efficiency of gas exchange.[15]

Along with these changes in the lung, there are important changes in the upper airway. There is a loss of muscular pharyngeal support, making the elderly more susceptible to upper airway obstruction.[15] There is also a decrease in respiratory effort in response to upper airway occlusion.[15] Protective mechanisms of coughing and swallowing also diminish with time, making geriatric individuals more at risk for aspiration.[15] A presumed explanation for these changes includes peripheral differentiation along with decreased central nervous system reflex activity.[15]

These changes in the respiratory system (see **Table 3**) contribute to the pulmonary complications that can be seen after anesthesia.[15] The decrease in chest wall compliance results in an increase in geriatric patients' work of breathing after anesthesia.[15] The changes in lung mechanics impair geriatric patients' gas exchange and the tendency for small airway closure leading to atelectasis.[15] Several studies have shown that age alone is a significant independent predictor of risk for perioperative pulmonary complications.[15]

GASTROINTESTINAL SYSTEM

Age-related changes occur along most of the gastrointestinal track (**Table 4**). There is a decrease in the amplitude of esophageal contractions and a decrease in the number of peristaltic waves that occur with a standard swallow.[19] One study found an increase in the number of disordered contractions in the body of the esophagus.[19] Geriatric individuals are also subject to prolonged gastric emptying.[19] One study showed that a standard mixed meal took double the time to empty compared with younger subjects.[19] Thus, elderly patients are at higher risk for aspiration at anesthetic induction or in the postoperative period. Gastric acid secretion decreases with age at both a basal rate and when fixed doses of exogenous gastrin are given to stimulate production.[19] This process is secondary to the development of atrophic gastritis, which causes a decrease in secretion of acid and intrinsic factor (but not enough to result

Table 4 Changes in the gastrointestinal and hepatic system with age			
Gastrointestinal Changes		**Hepatic Changes**	
Esophageal motility	▼	Hepatic blood flow	▼
Gastric acid secretion	▼	Hepatic volume	▼
Gastric emptying time	▲	Microsomal demethylation pathway	▼
Small intestine surface area	▼	Drug metabolism	▼

▲, Augmented; ▼, diminished.

in vitamin B_{12} malabsorption and pernicious anemia).[19] Atrophic gastritis may affect calcium bioavailability because of a limited ability to dissociate from food complexes.[19]

Pancreatic function does not seem to be diminished with age because there does not seem to be any diminished response to stimulation by secretin or cholecystokinin.[19] The mucosal surface of the small intestine is slightly diminished with aging.[19] Despite this, the ratio of mean surface area to volume of jejunal mucosa does not change with age.[19]

The liver experiences significant change with age (see **Table 4**). There is a reduction of liver volume, ranging from 20% to 40% across the human lifespan.[2,20] With the loss of volume, there is also age-related decline in hepatic blood flow.[2,20] The age-related loss of endoplasmic reticulum surface causes a strong negative correlation between age and hepatic microsomal phase-I drug metabolizing activity.[2,20] This decline in total capacity of the liver to metabolize drugs can increase the incidence of adverse drug reactions.[20] This decline can be very variable, from drug to drug and from person to person.[20]

RENAL AND VOLUME REGULATION SYSTEM

Renal function declines related to age have been well documented within multiple geographic settings and patient populations and by using a wide range of methods and parameters (**Table 5**).[21] There is a cumulative increase in patients with end-stage renal disease with increasing age.[22] Age-related renal decline is affected by gender, with men more affected than women secondary to increased damage from vascular changes and androgen production.[21] Aging causes both creatinine clearance and glomerular filtration rates to decline, resulting in not only a sharp increase in chronic renal impairment and end-stage renal failure but increased susceptibility to acute insults.[21]

Electrolyte homeostasis is also affected with age. There is a slower homeostatic responsiveness to sodium changes and a decreased ability to maximally dilute or

Table 5 Changes in the renal system with age			
Number of nephrons	▼	Tubular secretions	▼
Glomerular filtration rate	▼	Ability to conserve sodium	▼
Renal blood flow	▼	Total body water	▼
Ability to concentrate urine	▼	Thirst perception	▼

▲, Augmented; ▼, diminished.

concentrate urine.[21,23] There is also a global impairment of movement of other electrolytes and transport of ions across the tubular epithelium.[21]

There are significant changes to the renal vascular network in the geriatric population, including a reduction in the actual and proportional renal blood flow with age.[21] After the fourth decade, there is a 10% decrease in renal blood flow with each decade thereafter.[23] With this diminished renal blood flow, there is an accompanying decrease in responsiveness and autoregulation of volume status.[21] The intrarenal arterial changes are similar to the systemic changes: arteriolosclerosis, intimal hypertrophy, and medial hypertrophy.[21]

There are also significant interstitial changes to an aging kidney. The size of the kidney increases to the fifth decade and then starts to decrease.[21] This volume loss is thought to be caused by tubule-interstitial changes, including infarction, scaring, and fibrosis, resulting in decreased clearance capabilities.[21]

The renin-angiotensin-aldosterone system is also affected with age, resulting in substantial declines in plasma renin activity.[24] The most significant decreases are found from the sixth decade onward.[24] Age has a greater effect on the decrease in plasma renin and aldosterone level compared with angiotensin II.[24]

Geriatric patients have pharmacokinetic changes in the absorption, distribution, metabolism, and excretion of anesthetic drugs.[22] There is a reduction in systemic clearance of drugs that are eliminated unchanged by the kidney caused by age-related changes in glomerular filtration rate and tubular function.[22] There is also a higher incidence of chronic kidney disease; along with the diminished blood flow and changes to autoregulation, this leads to an increase in prevalence of perioperative acute kidney injury.[21,22]

ENDOCRINE SYSTEM

There is a decline in endocrine function with age that includes decreased tissue responsiveness and a reduction in hormone secretion from peripheral glands (**Table 6**).[25] Examples include reductions in thyroid-stimulating hormone and triiodothyronine (T3). Age also results in a dampening of circadian hormonal and nonhormonal rhythms.[25]

Impaired glucose tolerance develops in more than 50% of individuals older than 80 years of age.[26] There is a decrease in insulin production by beta cells, an increase in insulin resistance related to poor diet, an increase in abdominal fat mass, and a decrease in lean body mass. These changes all contribute to the deterioration of glucose metabolism[26] and make elderly patients at higher risk of poor glycemic control in the perioperative setting.

Women typically experience menopause in the sixth decade of life when serum estradiol concentrations are lower and follicle-stimulating hormone concentrations are higher than in younger women.[25] Luteinizing hormone does not change like

Table 6 Changes in the endocrine system with age			
Muscle mass	▼	Male testosterone levels	▼
Fat mass	▲	Male follicle-stimulating hormone	▲
Female estradiol	▼	Male luteinizing hormone	▲
Female follicle-stimulating hormone	▲	Serum thyroxine (T4)	■
Female luteinizing hormone	■	Serum triiodothyronine (T3)	▼

▲ augmented; ▼ diminished; ■ unchanged.

follicle-stimulating hormone.[25] These changes, along with the decrease of estrogen levels, increase the risk of cardiovascular events, rapid loss of skeletal mass, vasomotor instability, psychological symptoms, and atrophy of estrogen-responsive tissue.[25]

Male gonadal steroid production also changes with age; a change termed andropause.[25] There is a marked decline in free testosterone levels from an increase in sex hormone–binding globulin levels.[25] The age of this decline is variable, and the physiologic consequences are unclear.[25] There is also a decline in total serum testosterone concentrations caused by a decrease in production rates as men age.[25]

SUMMARY

No matter the mechanism, aging affects the physiology of every major organ system. The nervous system experiences cognitive decline and volume loss. The cardiovascular system changes result in lower cardiac output and higher blood pressures leading to significant changes to the structure and function of the heart. The respiratory system changes lead to impaired oxygenation, diminished ventilation/perfusion matching, and an increased risk of atelectasis. The gastrointestinal system experiences a delay in emptying along with diminished hepatic metabolism. The renal system changes result in a diminished glomerular filtration rate and a diminished ability to control electrolyte hemostasis. The endocrine system results in hormonal changes that lead to variation in the patients' conditions. Importantly, all these changes can have major effects on the perioperative course of a geriatric patient, and anesthesia providers require an understanding of these changes and how they will affect the management of their geriatric patients.

REFERENCES

1. Maguire SL, Slater BMJ. Physiology of ageing. Anaesth Intensive Care Med 2013; 14:310–2.
2. Schmucker DL. Age-related changes in liver structure and function: implications for disease? Exp Gerontol 2005;40:650–9.
3. Rooke GA. Cardiovascular aging and anesthetic implications. J Cardiothorac Vasc Anesth 2003;17:512–23.
4. Priebe HJ. The aged cardiovascular risk patient. Br J Anaesth 2000;85:763–78.
5. Small SA. Age-related memory decline: current concepts and future directions. Arch Neurol 2001;58:360–4.
6. Peters R. Ageing and the brain. Postgrad Med J 2006;82:84–8.
7. Trollor JN, Valenzuela MJ. Brain ageing in the new millennium. Aust N Z J Psychiatry 2001;35:788–805.
8. Farrall AJ, Wardlaw JM. Blood-brain barrier: ageing and microvascular disease–systematic review and meta-analysis. Neurobiol Aging 2009;30:337–52.
9. Abbott NJ, Ronnback L, Hansson E. Astrocyte-endothelial interactions at the blood-brain barrier. Nat Rev Neurosci 2006;7:41–53.
10. Sharshar T, Hopkinson NS, Orlikowski D, et al. Science review: the brain in sepsis–culprit and victim. Crit Care 2005;9:37–44.
11. Brown EN, Purdon PL. The aging brain and anesthesia. Curr Opin Anaesthesiol 2013;26:414–9.
12. Ungvari Z, Kaley G, de Cabo R, et al. Mechanisms of vascular aging: new perspectives. J Gerontol A Biol Sci Med Sci 2010;65:1028–41.
13. Bursi F, Weston SA, Redfield MM, et al. Systolic and diastolic heart failure in the community. JAMA 2006;296:2209–16.

14. Dai DF, Rabinovitch PS, Ungvari Z. Mitochondria and cardiovascular aging. Circ Res 2012;110:1109–24.
15. Sprung J, Gajic O, Warner DO. Review article: age related alterations in respiratory function - anesthetic considerations. Can J Anaesth 2006;53:1244–57.
16. Vaz Fragoso CA, Gill TM. Respiratory impairment and the aging lung: a novel paradigm for assessing pulmonary function. J Gerontol A Biol Sci Med Sci 2012;67:264–75.
17. Chan ED, Welsh CH. Geriatric respiratory medicine. Chest 1998;114:1704–33.
18. Sharma G, Goodwin J. Effect of aging on respiratory system physiology and immunology. Clin Interv Aging 2006;1:253–60.
19. Russell RM. Changes in gastrointestinal function attributed to aging. Am J Clin Nutr 1992;55:1203S–7S.
20. Schmucker DL. Aging and the liver: an update. J Gerontol A Biol Sci Med Sci 1998;53:B315–20.
21. Martin JE, Sheaff MT. Renal ageing. J Pathol 2007;211:198–205.
22. Silva FG. The aging kidney: a review–part II. Int Urol Nephrol 2005;37:419–32.
23. Silva FG. The aging kidney: a review – part I. Int Urol Nephrol 2005;37:185–205.
24. Epstein M. Aging and the kidney. J Am Soc Nephrol 1996;7:1106–22.
25. Chahal HS, Drake WM. The endocrine system and ageing. J Pathol 2007;211: 173–80.
26. Lamberts SW, van den Beld AW, van der Lely AJ. The endocrinology of aging. Science 1997;278:419–24.

Geriatric Pharmacology

Shamsuddin Akhtar, MD*, Ramachandran Ramani, MD

KEYWORDS

- Geriatric • Pharmacology • Anesthetics • Aging

KEY POINTS

- Anesthetizing elderly patients requires understanding of the pharmacokinetic and pharmacodynamic changes with aging.
- Practitioners need to recognize the effect of administering multiple anesthetics and their interactions with nonanesthetic medications.
- Neurologic changes with aging can affect anesthesia.
- Older patients show more hypotension and greater hemodynamic lability during anesthesia.
- Elderly patients require much less anesthetic.

INTRODUCTION

The aging process is characterized by a significant level of complexity, which makes the perioperative care of the elderly patients extremely challenging. Typically, elderly patients have multiple morbidities and are often taking multiple medications.[1–3] Polypharmacy is the norm in the elderly.[2] Effects of drug interactions are substantially magnified with advanced age. It is also well recognized that sicker patients require less anesthetic. Frequently, elderly patients also have geriatric syndromes; for example, falls, malnutrition, delirium, and mild cognitive dysfunction.[4,5] Against this background of reduced reserve (frailty), multimorbidity, and polypharmacy, geriatric patients present for surgical and anesthetic care.

Elderly patients require less anesthetic, which is often attributed to progressive pharmacokinetic and pharmacodynamic changes that occur with aging. Although pharmacokinetic changes have been well characterized, the data are typically from healthy elderly patients (American Society of Anesthesiologists [ASA] I/II) or patients who are less than 80 years old.[6] Most of the pharmacologic data are extrapolated to older octogenarians and nonagenarians.

Anesthetizing very elderly patients requires understanding of the pharmacokinetic and pharmacodynamic changes with aging. Practitioners also need to recognize the

Department of Anesthesiology, Yale University School of Medicine, 333 Cedar Street, Tompkins # 3, New Haven, CT 06520, USA
* Corresponding author.
E-mail address: shamsuddin.akhtar@yale.edu

Anesthesiology Clin 33 (2015) 457–469
http://dx.doi.org/10.1016/j.anclin.2015.05.004   anesthesiology.theclinics.com
1932-2275/15/$ – see front matter © 2015 Elsevier Inc. All rights reserved.

effect of simultaneously administering multiple anesthetics and their interactions with nonanesthetic medications. This article addresses current understanding of mechanisms of general anesthesia, neurologic changes with aging that can affect anesthesia, and commonly accepted pharmacokinetic and pharmacodynamics changes with aging. It also discusses specific commonly used drugs, the impact of combining and overdosing elderly patients, and concludes with recommendations for dosing elderly patients and future areas of research.

CEREBRAL MECHANISMS OF GENERAL ANESTHESIA

Cellular and molecular mechanisms underlying induction of general anesthesia are well understood. All anesthetic agents are similar in decreasing neuronal firing, either through the enhancement of inhibitory currents or the reduction of excitatory currents within the brain.[7,8] Gamma-aminobutyric acid type A ($GABA_A$) and N-methyl-D-aspartate (NMDA) receptors in the cortex, thalamus, brainstem, and striatum seem to be the most important targets of anesthesia.[9,10] Activation of these receptor targets of general anesthetics cause either enhancement of inhibitory currents mediated by GABA and glycine protein channels, or reductions of excitatory currents mediated by glutamate and acetylcholine protein channels, and enhancement of background potassium leak currents.[8] Barbiturates, etomidate, propofol, and benzodiazepines target $GABA_A$ receptors, the main inhibitory receptors in the brain, expressed in nearly one-third of all synapses.[9,11] Reduction of excitatory neurotransmitter receptors by anesthetics contributes to inactivation of large regions of the brain, thus resulting in a neurodepressive effect of anesthetics and unconsciousness.[9] Glutamate, the major excitatory neurotransmitter in the brain, activates 2 subclasses of receptors: the NMDA receptors and the non-NMDA receptors, which are further divided into a-amino-3-hydroxy-5-methyl-4-isoxazole propionic acid and kainate receptors.[12] The activation of NMDA receptors necessitates binding of glutamate and either glycine or D-serine.[13] Volatile anesthetics, xenon, and nitrous oxide inhibit NMDA receptor activity.[14–16] Xenon has a minimal or no effect on the $GABA_A$ ligand channels. Ketamine inhibits NMDA-mediated glutamatergic inputs with an excitatory activity in the cortex and limbic system, ultimately leading to unconsciousness.[13]

Given that nearly all anesthetics decrease global cerebral metabolism in a dose-dependent manner, it was generally accepted that a general (eg, nonspecific) reduction in metabolism was the common mechanism for producing anesthesia-induced loss of consciousness.[17] However, newer research using electroencephalogram (EEG), functional MRI, and other imaging techniques has shown that unconsciousness is more complicated than simple global depression.[7,13] Different regions of the brain are intricately connected to each other and are constantly communicating with each other. The human brain has a highly organized network of communication pathways between functionally related regions.[18,19] This network is also called connectivity, which executes the basic functions of the brain. Functional connectivity refers to the temporal correlations between different related regions of the brain, linked to functionally related neurophysiologic events. It is this inherent functional connectivity that sustains a conscious state. Various functional networks in the brain have been identified. The default mode network (DMN) is one such network whose function has been explored in many studies.[20] The anterior part of the DMN is the prefrontal cortex. During the process of development, the frontal lobe is the last part of the brain to get myelinated, and during senescence it is the first part where demyelination occurs. It is active in the resting state. In contrast, when a task is being performed there is a decrease in activity in the DMN. The more challenging the task, the greater is the deactivation of DMN. This decrease in DMN activity during the execution of a task helps shift attention and focus on the task. In elderly people there is a decrease in activity in the DMN in the resting state and the ability to decrease DMN activity during a task is less.[21,22] It is this change in DMN function that results in inability to quickly change focus and difficulty in dual task performance in elderly people. Executive function is also impaired in the elderly for the same reason. In addition to a decrease in activity with aging in the DMN, there is a difference between anterior and posterior regions of the network. The neuronal activity in the anterior part of the DMN decreases more than the activity in the posterior of the network with aging. There is a correlation between chronologic age, activity in the anterior part of the DMN, and cognition.

Anesthetics modify functional connectivity within and between resting-state cortical networks. Although anesthetics clinically cause generalized unconsciousness, the effects of anesthetic agents differ in their specific regions of the brain and networks.[13] For example, the intravenous anesthetic propofol preferentially suppresses activity within the frontoparietal cortex, as does the inhalational anesthetic sevoflurane.[23] The thalamus is a second site of action for most anesthetics, and it was accepted that the thalamus was the primary region mediating loss of consciousness during anesthesia. However, newer studies show that the decreased thalamic activity during induction of anesthesia follows both cortical depression and loss of consciousness. Although there are some inconsistencies in the different studies, the prevalent view is that unconsciousness during anesthesia arises as a consequence of the disruption of corticocortical connections.[24] Under anesthesia, decreased corticocortical connectivity has been reported in various higher-order brain networks, including the DMN and the executive control network.[25,26] It is now widely held that the cortex is the primary site of anesthetic action, whereas subcortical structures are suppressed secondary to decreased excitatory corticothalamic feedback.[27] With deepening anesthetic-induced sedation, sensory information processing in cortex is sequentially impaired from more to less complex, in a dose-dependent manner. Brain activation declines first in higher-order, or association, cortices before responses in primary cortical areas are attenuated. In contrast, recovery of consciousness following anesthesia is accompanied by the restoration of functional coupling between lower-order areas, including subcortical and limbic regions, and frontal and inferior parietal cortices.[28]

To date, increased sensitivity to anesthetics in the elderly has been attributed to loss of neuronal tissue or poorly defined changes in receptor functions. Progressive changes in functional connectivity with aging and varying effects of anesthetics provide another explanation for increased sensitivity in the elderly. In addition to anesthetic toxicity, it may also explain the mechanism behind the cognitive dysfunction that is associated with anesthetics.

PHARMACOKINETIC CHANGES WITH AGING
Body Composition

Pharmacokinetics of anesthetic agents are affected by progressive physiologic changes that occur with aging. Total body water decreases by 10% to 15% in the elderly.[29] A decrease in total body water causes a decrease in the measured central compartment volume in the elderly. This decrease can lead to increase in initial plasma concentrations following rapid intravenous administration of anesthetics. Body fat increases by 20% to 40% as muscle mass decreases progressively with aging. Thus lipid-soluble drugs (most of the intravenous anesthetics) have large volumes of distribution, with potential to prolong the clinical effect of a given medication.

Changes in serum proteins include a decrease in plasma albumin and a slight increase in alpha-1 acid glycoprotein. Although theoretically these changes can affect circulating free drug concentrations and subsequently affect the concentration of drug at the effect site (ke0), in practice they do not seem to have an important impact on geriatric anesthetic pharmacology.[30] Of bigger concern is the lack of adjustment for lean body mass and weight in drug dosing in the elderly.

Metabolism

Hepatic blood flow declines by 10% per decade, and liver mass decreases by 20% to 40% in elderly people.[31] Drugs that are metabolized by microsomal cytochrome P450 enzymes may be affected. In general, these changes result in reduction in the clearance of flow-limited drugs by about 30% to 40%, which corresponds with a decrease in hepatic blood flow, but there is no alteration for capacity-limited drugs.

Various aspects of renal function also decline with normal aging.[32,33] The salient changes that accompany normal renal aging are as follows:

1. Renal mass progressively declines with aging.
2. Renal vascular dysautonomy: this term reflects attenuation of the autonomic renal vascular reflexes to protect the kidney from hypotensive or hypertensive states.
3. Senile hypofiltration: this term describes progressive decline in glomerular filtration rate (GFR) at about 1 mL/y after 30 years, which is seen in about two-thirds of the elderly.
4. Tubular dysfunction, which leads to the reduction in maximal tubular capacity to reabsorb and excrete solutes, especially sodium.
5. Medullary hypotonicity: this phenomenon describes lower tonicity of the renal medulla in the elderly compared with younger individuals, which causes reduced effect of antidiuretic hormone and, as a consequence, a reduction in water absorption. Elderly patients are unable to concentrate or dilute urine to the maximum.
6. Tubular frailty: this term refers to renal tubular cells being more susceptible to hypoxic or nephrotoxicity injury and taking longer to recover from acute tubular necrosis.

The clinical consequences of these changes are profound. The aging kidney is more susceptible to injury, less able to accommodate hemodynamic changes, and it is also not able to manage water and salt perturbations. Low GFR and diminished tubular function lead to reduced ability to concentrate urine, which means that the obligatory urinary volume to excrete waste products also needs to increase. In contrast, because of decreased GFR, the ability to excrete access free water is diminished, making the elderly prone to fluid overload and pulmonary edema. Elderly people are more vulnerable to develop hypo-osmolar states (hyponatremia) if large amounts of hypo-osmolar fluids are administered. Extravascular volume overload is a significant risk in elderly patients. Neuromuscular blockers that are excreted renally should be carefully dosed in the elderly.

PHARMACOLOGIC CONSIDERATIONS OF SPECIFIC ANESTHETIC MEDICATIONS
Inhalational Anesthetics

The minimum alveolar concentration (MAC) required to achieve adequate anesthetic depth progressively decreases with age. By some estimates, MAC values decrease by 6% per decade after 40 years for volatile anesthetics and about 7.7% per decade for nitrous oxide.[34] The pharmacodynamic correlate for increased volatile anesthetic and nitrous oxide sensitivity in the elderly is unknown but it may be related to progressive changes in functional connectivity in the elderly. The effect of volatile anesthetics is additive. Thus, an 80-year-old patient who is on 66% nitrous oxide requires only 0.3% sevoflurane to achieve 1 MAC anesthetic concentration (**Fig. 1**). The hemodynamic impact of excessive anesthetic administration is well recognized.

Propofol

Propofol activates the $GABA_A$ receptors and hyperpolarizes the cell membrane. Functionally, propofol induces loss of consciousness by decreasing the activity in the DMN, other higher mental function networks, and the auditory network.[25,26] Some studies have shown that the posterior part of the DMN (precuneus, posterior cingulate, and inferior parietal lobe) is more sensitive to propofol than the anterior part.[14,35] The pharmacology of propofol is significantly altered with aging. Both pharmacodynamics and pharmacokinetic aspects of propofol pharmacology are affected.[15,16] Age-related changes have been found for both induction doses and infusions. In one study, half-maximal effective concentration (EC_{50}) values for loss of consciousness were 2.35, 1.8, and 1.25 μg/mL in healthy volunteers who were 20, 50, and 75 years old, respectively.[15] This finding reflects a nearly 50% decrease in dosing. For the same fixed dose of anesthesia, elderly patients developed deeper EEG stages, needed more time to reach deeper anesthetic stages (as determined by EEG), and also required more time for recovery.[36] Older patients also needed less propofol for steady-state maintenance, for a defined stage of hypnosis as detected by EEG, than the younger patients (5.9 ± 1.7 mg/kg for patients <50 years old, vs 3.5 ± 1.4 mg mg of those older than 70 years).[37] For the same plasma concentration of propofol, the reduction in blood pressure with propofol administration is significantly greater in the elderly than in young patients.[38] Infusing a bolus over a longer period of time can minimize this greater hemodynamic effect of propofol in the elderly.

Clearance and volume of central compartment decreases for propofol with age. Furthermore, there are gender differences in propofol pharmacokinetics. Propofol clearance is considerably more decreased in women than in men.[39] Propofol infusion rates required to achieve a persistent level of moderate sedation are lower in the elderly. Current literature suggests a 20% reduction in the induction dose of propofol and some investigators have recommended doses as low as 0.8 to 1.2 mg/kg in elderly patients.[38,40] Although the drug has been extensively studied, the investigations have been limited to healthy older patients. In one landmark study, elderly patients were not administered more than 1 mg/kg for induction for safety reasons.[14] Similarly, in a study analyzing 21 previously published data sets on the anesthetic induction agent propofol (660 patients in total) only 6 patients were more than 80 years old.[6] Practitioners should recognize that the current practice for anesthetic care of the very elderly is based on extrapolation from younger, and healthier, patients.

Etomidate

Etomidate is an anesthetic and amnestic, but not an analgesic. It is considered an ideal drug in an elderly because it is associated with less hemodynamic instability than propofol or thiopental. However, a smaller initial volume of distribution and reduced clearance in the elderly, as well as a significant increase in anesthetic sensitivity, have been shown. Like propofol, much lower induction doses are recommended in the elderly. Elderly patients require 0.2 mg/kg for induction, as opposed to 0.3 to 0.4 mg/kg for young adults.

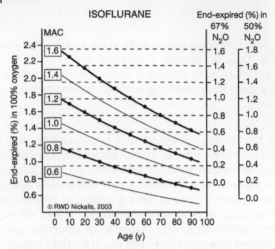

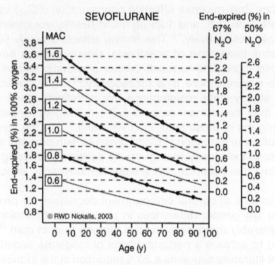

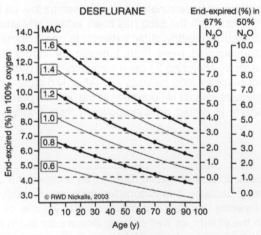

Fig. 1. Iso-MAC chart for isoflurane, sevoflurane, and desflurane. (*From* Nickalls RW, Mapleson WW. Age-related iso-MAC charts for isoflurane, sevoflurane and desflurane in man. Br J Anaesth 2003;91:170–4; with permission.)

Thiopental

In contrast with propofol, older studies (in which populations were limited to patients who were <80 years old) have shown no significant age-related changes in thiopental brain responsiveness or pharmacodynamics.[41] However, central volume of distribution of thiopental decreases in the elderly and total induction dose needs to be reduced. An optimal dose in an 80-year-old patient was suggested to be 2.5 mg/kg, which is 50% to 80% of the dose needed for an adult patient (3–5 mg/kg). Recovery after a bolus dose of thiopental is also delayed in older patients, because of decreased central volume of distribution.

Midazolam

Elderly patients are significantly more sensitive to midazolam than younger patients, primarily because of pharmacodynamics differences.[42] However, the exact mechanism of this pharmacodynamic difference is not known. Furthermore, the duration of effect may last much longer and can potentially contribute to postoperative delirium. Benzodiazepines should be avoided in elderly patients.[43] In addition, pharmacokinetics of midazolam are significantly altered in elderly patients. Midazolam clearance is reduced in the elderly by as much as 30% because of loss of functional hepatic tissue and probably decreases in hepatic perfusion. Furthermore, midazolam is metabolized to a pharmacologically active metabolite, hydroxymidazolam, which is excreted by the kidneys and may accumulate in patients with diminished renal function. A 75% reduction in dose from a 20-year-old to a 90-year-old has been recommended.[40]

Opioids

Pharmacodynamic changes within the opioid receptor system have been noted with aging.[44] Receptor density, receptor affinity, and binding may change with aging. Although increased sensitivity to opioids is attributed to pharmacodynamics changes to the effect of opioids, age-related pharmacokinetic changes, especially opioid metabolite pharmacokinetic changes, affect the choice of opioids that are used in the elderly. The liver mainly metabolizes opioids and the kidneys excrete the metabolites. Metabolites of some opioids (codeine, morphine, meperidine) are pharmacologic active, accounting for both persistent analgesia and many side effects. The primary risk of opioids is respiratory depression, the incidence of which is markedly increased with age.[45]

Fentanyl
Fentanyl is a highly selective mu receptor agonist. Earlier studies suggested that terminal half-life of fentanyl was prolonged in the elderly. However, subsequent studies have not found a significant influence of aging on fentanyl pharmacokinetics. Age has a greater effect on fentanyl pharmacodynamics than on pharmacokinetics. The EC_{50} required for the suppression of EEG, which is a measure of fentanyl potency, was decreased by approximately 50% from ages 20 to 85 years,[46] suggesting a 50% increase in the potency of fentanyl in octogenarians. Elderly patients are significantly more sensitive to fentanyl and therefore should receive reduced intravenous doses. Fentanyl can be administered either through oral mucosa or transdermally. Although clearance of fentanyl is not affected, transdermal absorption of fentanyl is delayed in the elderly.[47]

Remifentanil
Remifentanil is an ultrashort-acting synthetic opioid and is metabolized by nonspecific tissue and plasma esterases. This property makes it an ideal drug for use in the elderly

because it has a short half-life and does not depend on liver and renal function, which are affected with aging. Remifentanil pharmacology has been well studied in different age groups. In one study, the volume of the central compartment decreased by approximately 25% and clearance decreased by 33% from the ages of 20 to 85 years. Elderly patients are also more sensitive to remifentanil. The EC_{50} and plasma effect-site equilibration constant decreased by approximately 50% over the age range of 20 to 85 years. The onset and offset of remifentanil are also slower in elderly individuals, although the blood concentrations were similar to those of younger patients. The peak drug effect after a bolus injection occurred at 2 to 3 minutes in elderly patients, as opposed to the expected effect in about 90 seconds in younger individuals. Elderly individuals need about half of the bolus dose than younger individuals need for the same drug effect. As with fentanyl and alfentanil, this is because of increased pharmacodynamic sensitivity in the elderly rather than pharmacokinetic changes. Elderly patients require an infusion rate about one-third that of younger people, because of the combined impact of increased sensitivity and decreased clearance.[48]

Meperidine

Meperidine is a weak mu agonist with only approximately 10% of the effectiveness of morphine. It is metabolized in the liver to normeperidine, which is excreted by the kidneys. The half-life of normeperidine is 15 to 30 hours and it can cause agitation and seizures at high concentrations. Meperidine also has negative inotropic properties and intrinsic anticholinergic properties, and its use has been associated with development of postoperative delirium in elderly patients.[49] Meperidine is not recommended in elderly patients except in very small doses to manage postoperative shivering.

Neuromuscular Blocking Drugs

The pharmacodynamics of neuromuscular blocking drugs are not significantly altered with age. Studies of the relationship between depth of neuromuscular blockade and plasma with concentration show little if any difference with age. The effective-dose in 95% of the population (ED_{95}) of neuromuscular blocking is essentially the same for young and old patients. In contrast, the pharmacokinetics of neuromuscular drugs are significantly altered with age. The onset to maximal block may be delayed by 30 seconds to a minute. Because these drugs are metabolized by the liver and excreted by the kidney, hepatic and renal dysfunction can significantly prolong their effects. The recovery time from the neuromuscular blockade could be increased by 50%.[50] Furthermore, the impact of residual neuromuscular blockade (0.7–0.8 train of 4 ratios) on pharyngeal function can be significant in the elderly.[51] Because cisatracurium does not depend on hepatic or renal function for clearance, it is considered the neuromuscular blocker of choice for the elderly.[50]

APPLYING PHARMACOLOGIC KNOWLEDGE TO PRACTICE

Based on the information presented earlier it is clear that requirements of most anesthetics decrease by 25% to 75% with aging. Balanced anesthesia is considered a standard in contemporary anesthetic practice. However, the synergistic effect of multiple anesthetics, although acknowledged, has not been extensively studied and is practically nonexistent in ASA III/IV elderly patients. Propofol and midazolam are known to have hemodynamic effects that result in decreases in arterial blood pressure,[52] and coadministration of these two drugs has a synergistic effect.[53] Fentanyl, when used as the sole or primary induction agent, has been shown to result in hemodynamic stability, although it can lead to prolonged ventilation. However, studies have shown that when used in combination with propofol, opioids reduce the plasma propofol concentration required for loss of consciousness.[54,55] Specifically, alfentanil has been shown to enhance the depressant effects of propofol on systolic blood pressure. Hemodynamic stability therefore does not seem to be improved with combinations of propofol and alfentanil.[55] Studies combining midazolam, propofol, and fentanyl show a synergistic effect of these drugs, which is reflected by significant reductions in propofol dose requirement when adding midazolam pretreatment to a standard propofol and fentanyl induction. This synergistic effect seemed to be even more significant in the older age group (>60 years).[56] Although this study did not determine each induction agent's individual effect on blood pressure, the postinduction hemodynamic changes seen in this study are likely in part to be caused by the synergistic action of the induction agents used, and this effect is likely more significant in the elderly.

Practitioners are aware that elderly patients require much less anesthetic, however, the extent of anesthetic requirement is frequently underappreciated. Preliminary results of our study suggest that although practitioners do reduce the induction dosing of propofol in the elderly, they still administer the upper limit of recommended doses (personal observations). Practitioners are also more likely to correct for severity of illness (ie, the ASA class) than age in patients undergoing gastrointestinal endoscopic procedures.[57]

CONSEQUENCES OF OVERDOSING ANESTHETICS IN ELDERLY PATIENTS

Older patients are known to show more hypotension and greater lability during anesthesia than young adults.[58,59] It is also well known that induction of anesthesia by bolus administration of propofol can produce significant hypotension.[60] There is evidence that hypotension and hypertension during general anesthesia are independently associated with adverse outcomes in patients having both noncardiac and cardiac surgery.[61–64] Although the consequences of postinduction hypotension are not entirely known, Reich and colleagues[64] noted in a retrospective review that 9% of their patients experienced severe hypotension 0 to 10 minutes after induction of general anesthesia. The patients with postinduction hypotension were more likely to experience prolonged postoperative stays and/or death than those patients without postinduction hypotension (13.3% vs 8.6%).[61] A prospective cohort study by Monk and colleagues[61] also showed that 1-year mortality risk was increased with longer duration of intraoperative hypotension, with a 0.36% increase in mortality risk per minute that the mean arterial pressure was less than 80 mm Hg. More recently, Walsh and colleagues[62] found that patients with intraoperative hypotension in which the mean arterial pressure decreased to less than 55 mm Hg had an increased risk for both acute kidney injury and myocardial injury. Even short durations (1–5 minutes) of hypotension were associated with an increased risk for these adverse outcomes; however the risk increased with increased duration of intraoperative hypotension.

The elderly population is especially at risk for postinduction hypotension given the pathophysiologic cardiovascular changes associated with aging. There is decreased baroreceptor sensitivity with increasing age, which impairs the ability to buffer short-term changes in blood pressure. Decreased responsiveness to beta-adrenoreceptors and renin-angiotensin-aldosterone system stimulation also increases the risk for hypotension in older patients.[65] Given the increased risk of both morbidity and mortality associated with even short durations of postinduction hypotension, careful management of anesthetic dosing and hemodynamics in the elderly could improve the postoperative outcomes for these patients.

SUMMARY

Aging involves changes in several physiologic processes that lead to decreased volumes of distribution, slowed metabolism, and increased end-organ sensitivity to anesthetic drugs. These changes generally result in increased potency. Although it is well known that elderly patients require significantly less anesthetic medication, the extent of reduction is underappreciated and not uniformly applied in practice. The impact of potential anesthetic drug overdosing on intermediate and long-term outcomes is not fully appreciated. Large database studies are beginning to show the consequences of even short-term hemodynamic perturbations in the perioperative period. These perturbations are probably of greater consequence in frail, elderly patients with reduced reserves. Dosing of anesthetics is under the control of anesthesiologists and the impact of anesthetic overdosing should be recognized. Just because hypotension can be treated readily with vasopressors and fluids, it does not mean that it should be allowable. Fluid therapy and vasopressor therapy have consequences and potentially contribute to morbidity in the elderly. Prevention is better than cure.

With the increasing population of patients more than 65 years of age, it may be necessary to think of age as a continuous variable when considering anesthetic drug dosing in older patients rather than thinking of adult versus elderly patients.

Little is known about the pharmacodynamic differences in people more than 85 years old,[66] and this is one of the fastest growing populations in the United States. Further pharmacologic studies are required in the elderly population (>85 years). Such studies will help to delineate the pharmacokinetic/pharmacodynamic differences in this population beyond what has been studied for those patients more than 65 years of age. Practice of anesthesia, though very safe, can still be improved for this vulnerable population.

REFERENCES

1. Boyd CM, Kent DM. Evidence-based medicine and the hard problem of multimorbidity. J Gen Intern Med 2014;29:552–3.
2. Wehling M. Guideline-driven polypharmacy in elderly, multimorbid patients is basically flawed: there are almost no guidelines for these patients. J Am Geriatr Soc 2011;59:376–7.
3. Onder G, Landi F, Fusco D, et al. Recommendations to prescribe in complex older adults: results of the CRIteria to assess appropriate Medication use among Elderly complex patients (CRIME) project. Drugs Aging 2014;31:33–45.
4. Xue QL. The frailty syndrome: definition and natural history. Clin Geriatr Med 2011;27:1–15.
5. Turner G, Clegg A. Best practice guidelines for the management of frailty: a British Geriatrics Society, Age UK and Royal College of General Practitioners report. Age Ageing 2014;43:744–7.
6. Eleveld DJ, Proost JH, Cortinez LI, et al. A general purpose pharmacokinetic model for propofol. Anesth Analg 2014;118:1221–37.
7. MacDonald AA, Naci L, MacDonald PA, et al. Anesthesia and neuroimaging: investigating the neural correlates of unconsciousness. Trends Cogn Sci 2015; 19:100–7.
8. Franks NP. Molecular targets underlying general anaesthesia. Br J Pharmacol 2006;147(Suppl 1):S72–81.
9. Franks NP. General anaesthesia: from molecular targets to neuronal pathways of sleep and arousal. Nat Rev Neurosci 2008;9:370–86.

10. Campagna JA, Miller KW, Forman SA. Mechanisms of actions of inhaled anesthetics. N Engl J Med 2003;348:2110–24.

11. Kopp Lugli A, Yost CS, Kindler CH. Anaesthetic mechanisms: update on the challenge of unravelling the mystery of anaesthesia. Eur J Anaesthesiol 2009;26:807–20.

12. Cull-Candy S, Brickley S, Farrant M. NMDA receptor subunits: diversity, development and disease. Curr Opin Neurobiol 2001;11:327–35.

13. Uhrig L, Dehaene S, Jarraya B. Cerebral mechanisms of general anesthesia. Ann Fr Anesth Reanim 2014;33:72–82.

14. Cavanna AE, Trimble MR. The precuneus: a review of its functional anatomy and behavioural correlates. Brain 2006;129:564–83.

15. Schnider TW, Minto CF, Shafer SL, et al. The influence of age on propofol pharmacodynamics. Anesthesiology 1999;90:1502–16.

16. Vuyk J, Schnider T, Engbers F. Population pharmacokinetics of propofol for target-controlled infusion (TCI) in the elderly. Anesthesiology 2000;93:1557–60.

17. Alkire MT, Haier RJ, Shah NK, et al. Positron emission tomography study of regional cerebral metabolism in humans during isoflurane anesthesia. Anesthesiology 1997;86:549–57.

18. Biswal B, Yetkin FZ, Haughton VM, et al. Functional connectivity in the motor cortex of resting human brain using echo-planar MRI. Magn Reson Med 1995;34:537–41.

19. Raichle ME. The restless brain. Brain Connect 2011;1:3–12.

20. Raichle ME, MacLeod AM, Snyder AZ, et al. A default mode of brain function. Proc Natl Acad Sci U S A 2001;98:676–82.

21. Damoiseaux JS, Rombouts SA, Barkhof F, et al. Consistent resting-state networks across healthy subjects. Proc Natl Acad Sci U S A 2006;103:13848–53.

22. Grady CL, Springer MV, Hongwanishkul D, et al. Age-related changes in brain activity across the adult lifespan. J Cogn Neurosci 2006;18:227–41.

23. Kaisti KK, Langsjo JW, Aalto S, et al. Effects of sevoflurane, propofol, and adjunct nitrous oxide on regional cerebral blood flow, oxygen consumption, and blood volume in humans. Anesthesiology 2003;99:603–13.

24. Monti MM, Lutkenhoff ES, Rubinov M, et al. Dynamic change of global and local information processing in propofol-induced loss and recovery of consciousness. PLoS Comput Biol 2013;9:e1003271.

25. Jordan D, Ilg R, Riedl V, et al. Simultaneous electroencephalographic and functional magnetic resonance imaging indicate impaired cortical top-down processing in association with anesthetic-induced unconsciousness. Anesthesiology 2013;119:1031–42.

26. Boveroux P, Vanhaudenhuyse A, Bruno MA, et al. Breakdown of within- and between-network resting state functional magnetic resonance imaging connectivity during propofol-induced loss of consciousness. Anesthesiology 2010;113:1038–53.

27. Hudetz AG. General anesthesia and human brain connectivity. Brain Connect 2012;2:291–302.

28. Langsjo JW, Alkire MT, Kaskinoro K, et al. Returning from oblivion: imaging the neural core of consciousness. J Neurosci 2012;32:4935–43.

29. Beaufrere B, Morio B. Fat and protein redistribution with aging: metabolic considerations. Eur J Clin Nutr 2000;3(54 Suppl):S48–53.

30. Benet LZ, Hoener BA. Changes in plasma protein binding have little clinical relevance. Clin Pharmacol Ther 2002;71:115–21.

31. McLean AJ, Le Couteur DG. Aging biology and geriatric clinical pharmacology. Pharmacol Rev 2004;56:163–84.

32. Perico N, Remuzzi G, Benigni A. Aging and the kidney. Curr Opin Nephrol Hypertens 2011;20:312–7.
33. Karsch-Volk M, Schmid E, Wagenpfeil S, et al. Kidney function and clinical recommendations of drug dose adjustment in geriatric patients. BMC Geriatr 2013;13:92.
34. Nickalls RW, Mapleson WW. Age-related iso-MAC charts for isoflurane, sevoflurane and desflurane in man. Br J Anaesth 2003;91:170–4.
35. Xie G, Deschamps A, Backman SB, et al. Critical involvement of the thalamus and precuneus during restoration of consciousness with physostigmine in humans during propofol anaesthesia: a positron emission tomography study. Br J Anaesth 2011;106:548–57.
36. Schultz A, Grouven U, Zander I, et al. Age-related effects in the EEG during propofol anaesthesia. Acta Anaesthesiol Scand 2004;48:27–34.
37. Kreuer S, Schreiber JU, Bruhn J, et al. Impact of patient age on propofol consumption during propofol-remifentanil anaesthesia. Eur J Anaesthesiol 2005;22:123–8.
38. Kazama T, Ikeda K, Morita K, et al. Comparison of the effect-site k(eO)s of propofol for blood pressure and EEG bispectral index in elderly and younger patients. Anesthesiology 1999;90:1517–27.
39. White M, Kenny GN, Schraag S. Use of target controlled infusion to derive age and gender covariates for propofol clearance. Clin Pharmacokinet 2008;47:119–27.
40. Shafer SL. The pharmacology of anesthetic drugs in elderly patients. Anesthesiol Clin North America 2000;18:1–29, v.
41. Stanski DR, Maitre PO. Population pharmacokinetics and pharmacodynamics of thiopental: the effect of age revisited. Anesthesiology 1990;72:412–22.
42. Jacobs JR, Reves JG, Marty J, et al. Aging increases pharmacodynamic sensitivity to the hypnotic effects of midazolam. Anesth Analg 1995;80:143–8.
43. Barr J, Fraser GL, Puntillo K, et al. Clinical practice guidelines for the management of pain, agitation, and delirium in adult patients in the intensive care unit. Crit Care Med 2013;41:263–306.
44. Zubieta JK, Dannals RF, Frost JJ. Gender and age influences on human brain mu-opioid receptor binding measured by PET. Am J Psychiatry 1999;156:842–8.
45. Cepeda MS, Farrar JT, Baumgarten M, et al. Side effects of opioids during short-term administration: effect of age, gender, and race. Clin Pharmacol Ther 2003;74:102–12.
46. Scott JC, Ponganis KV, Stanski DR. EEG quantitation of narcotic effect: the comparative pharmacodynamics of fentanyl and alfentanil. Anesthesiology 1985;62:234–41.
47. Davis MP, Srivastava M. Demographics, assessment and management of pain in the elderly. Drugs Aging 2003;20:23–57.
48. Minto CF, Schnider TW, Egan TD, et al. Influence of age and gender on the pharmacokinetics and pharmacodynamics of remifentanil. I. Model development. Anesthesiology 1997;86:10–23.
49. Marcantonio ER, Juarez G, Goldman L, et al. The relationship of postoperative delirium with psychoactive medications. JAMA 1994;272:1518–22.
50. Ornstein E, Lien CA, Matteo RS, et al. Pharmacodynamics and pharmacokinetics of cisatracurium in geriatric surgical patients. Anesthesiology 1996;84:520–5.
51. Cedborg AI, Sundman E, Boden K, et al. Pharyngeal function and breathing pattern during partial neuromuscular block in the elderly: effects on airway protection. Anesthesiology 2014;120:312–25.

52. Vuyk J, Lichtenbelt BJ, Olofsen E, et al. Mixed-effects modeling of the influence of midazolam on propofol pharmacokinetics. Anesth Analg 2009;108:1522–30.
53. McClune S, McKay AC, Wright PM, et al. Synergistic interaction between midazolam and propofol. Br J Anaesth 1992;69:240–5.
54. Smith C, McEwan AI, Jhaveri R, et al. The interaction of fentanyl on the Cp50 of propofol for loss of consciousness and skin incision. Anesthesiology 1994;81: 820–8 [discussion: 26A].
55. Vuyk J, Engbers FH, Burm AG, et al. Pharmacodynamic interaction between propofol and alfentanil when given for induction of anesthesia. Anesthesiology 1996; 84:288–99.
56. Cressey DM, Claydon P, Bhaskaran NC, et al. Effect of midazolam pretreatment on induction dose requirements of propofol in combination with fentanyl in younger and older adults. Anaesthesia 2001;56:108–13.
57. Bing VZ, Heng J, Akhtar S. Anesthetic induction dosing in patients undergoing ambulatory gastrointestinal procedures: are we overdosing the elderly. American Society of Anesthesiologist, Annual Meeting, New Orleans, 2014;A3164.
58. Folkow B, Svanborg A. Physiology of cardiovascular aging. Physiol Rev 1993;73: 725–64.
59. Rooke GA. Cardiovascular aging and anesthetic implications. J Cardiothorac Vasc Anesth 2003;17:512–23.
60. Chan VW, Chung FF. Propofol infusion for induction and maintenance of anesthesia in elderly patients: recovery and hemodynamic profiles. J Clin Anesth 1996;8:317–23.
61. Monk TG, Saini V, Weldon BC, et al. Anesthetic management and one-year mortality after noncardiac surgery. Anesth Analg 2005;100:4–10.
62. Walsh M, Devereaux PJ, Garg AX, et al. Relationship between intraoperative mean arterial pressure and clinical outcomes after noncardiac surgery: toward an empirical definition of hypotension. Anesthesiology 2013;119:507–15.
63. Jain U, Laflamme CJ, Aggarwal A, et al. Electrocardiographic and hemodynamic changes and their association with myocardial infarction during coronary artery bypass surgery. A multicenter study. Multicenter Study of Perioperative Ischemia (McSPI) Research Group. Anesthesiology 1997;86:576–91.
64. Reich DL, Hossain S, Krol M, et al. Predictors of hypotension after induction of general anesthesia. Anesth Analg 2005;101:622–8 [table of contents].
65. Corcoran TB, Hillyard S. Cardiopulmonary aspects of anaesthesia for the elderly. Best Pract Res Clin Anaesthesiol 2011;25:329–54.
66. Bowie MW, Slattum PW. Pharmacodynamics in older adults: a review. Am J Geriatr Pharmacother 2007;5:263–303.

Preoperative Assessment of Geriatric Patients

Mariam Nakhaie, MD, Andrea Tsai, MD*

KEYWORDS

- Preoperative • Geriatric • Frailty • Nutritional status • Cardiovascular risk
- Pulmonary risk and complications • Medication history

KEY POINTS

- Guidelines recommend extensive neuropsychiatric evaluation and screening of geriatric patients in order to establish a baseline and to optimize perioperative care where possible.
- The new perioperative cardiac risk calculator is an interactive tool that more precisely quantifies risk based on the following 5 predictors: patient age, American Society of Anesthesiologists class and functional status, serum creatinine level, and type of surgery.
- Risk reduction strategies for postoperative pulmonary complications include medically optimizing the treatment of preexisting pulmonary disease, smoking cessation counseling, preoperative intensive inspiratory muscle training, and selective chest radiograph and pulmonary function testing.
- Frailty assessment is now recognized as an important component of the preoperative evaluation. Although no standardized test exists, there are several simple frailty assessment tools available to assist with documentation of frailty. Functional status has also been shown to have great prognostic ability for perioperative outcomes.
- Nutritional assessment of geriatric patients should be a key component of the preoperative evaluation because it can pinpoint areas of potential improvement before surgery. Poor nutritional status has been associated with worsened perioperative outcomes.
- The patient's prescription and nonprescription medications should be documented preoperatively and strong consideration should be given to discontinuation of nonessential medications to decrease the likelihood of medication interactions.

INTRODUCTION

The optimal preoperative assessment of geriatric patients has recently been outlined in a 2012 guideline by the American College of Surgeons (ACS) National Surgical Quality Improvement Program (NSQIP) and the American Geriatrics Society (AGS).[1] This is

Conflicts of Interest: The authors have no commercial or financial conflicts of interest.
Department of Anesthesiology, Tufts Medical Center, 800 Washington Street, Box 298, Boston, MA 02111, USA
* Corresponding author.
E-mail address: atsai@tuftsmedicalcenter.org

Anesthesiology Clin 33 (2015) 471–480
http://dx.doi.org/10.1016/j.anclin.2015.05.005 anesthesiology.theclinics.com

an important and timely publication because people aged 65 years and older represent a significant and growing proportion of the general as well as the surgical population and have an increased comorbidity prevalence and higher rates of perioperative complications even after controlling for comorbidities.[1,2] ACS NSQIP and AGS recommend a multisystem evaluation[1] (**Box 1**) that is detailed later, updated for more recent developments in system-specific recommendations.

NEUROPSYCHIATRIC EVALUATION

It is recommended that geriatric surgical patients have their cognitive ability, capacity for decision making, and risk factors for postoperative delirium assessed.[1] Furthermore, it is also recommended that they are screened for depression and alcohol and other substance abuse or dependence.[1] This neuropsychiatric assessment and screening serves multiple purposes: to establish a clinical baseline so that postoperative changes can be noted and potentially addressed; to guide optimal perioperative medical management; and to identify patients who, time permitting, can be further optimized before surgery.

To assess for cognitive impairment and dementia, the patient's prior history should be reviewed and knowledgeable informants (eg, family members) should be

---

Box 1
Checklist for the optimal preoperative assessment of geriatric surgical patients

In addition to conducting a complete history and physical examination of the patient, the following assessments are strongly recommended:

- Assess the patient's cognitive ability and capacity to understand the anticipated surgery.
- Screen the patient for depression.
- Identify the patient's risk factors for developing postoperative delirium.
- Screen for alcohol and other substance abuse/dependence.
- Perform a preoperative cardiac evaluation according to the American College of Cardiology/American Heart Association algorithm for patients undergoing noncardiac surgery.
- Identify the patient's risk factors for postoperative pulmonary complications and implement appropriate strategies for prevention.
- Document functional status and history of falls.
- Determine baseline frailty score.
- Assess the patient's nutritional status and consider preoperative interventions if the patient is at severe nutritional risk.
- Take an accurate and detailed medication history and consider appropriate perioperative adjustments. Monitor for polypharmacy.
- Determine the patient's treatment goals and expectations in the context of the possible treatment outcomes.
- Determine the patient's family and social support system.
- Order appropriate preoperative diagnostic tests focused on elderly patients.

From Chow WB, Rosenthal RA, Merkow RP, et al, American College of Surgeons National Surgical Quality Improvement Program, American Geriatrics Society. Optimal preoperative assessment of the geriatric surgical patient: a best practices guideline from the American College of Surgeons National Surgical Quality Improvement Program and the American Geriatrics Society. J Am Coll Surg 2012;215(4):454; with permission.

interviewed when available. In addition, guidelines also recommend the use of screening tools. The Mini-Cog, consisting of 3-item recall and clock drawing, has emerged as the most commonly recommended screening tool (**Box 2, Fig. 1**).[1,3] It is rapidly administered, requires little training to administer, is unbiased by variances in language and education, and is highly sensitive and specific for dementia detection.[3] Evidence of cognitive impairment helps to establish a baseline with which to compare postoperative changes and may prompt referral for further evaluation by a primary care physician or specialist. In addition, early detection of cognitive impairment sets an important context with which to interpret a patient's capacity, medication status, and functional status evaluation.

Capacity for decision making is practically and legally defined as possessing the ability to demonstrate 4 criteria: understanding, appreciation, reasoning, and choice. In order to have capacity, patients must be able to understand their treatment options, appreciate their clinical situation and consequences of choices, reason about the various options, and communicate a choice. Guidelines recommend that, before obtaining consent, surgeons should determine a geriatric patient's capacity. Approaches to this evaluation are outlined in **Table 1**.[4]

The most common postoperative complication in older adults is delirium, affecting up to 50% of older postoperative patients.[5] ACS NSQIP and AGS recommend that risk factors for delirium (**Box 3**) be identified and documented, and that efforts to avoid antihistamines and benzodiazepines be made in patients at increased risk for delirium.[1,5] A more comprehensive best practices statement regarding postoperative delirium was recently released by AGS and is an excellent resource and review of the subject.[5]

In addition, guidelines strongly recommend the preoperative screening of geriatric patients for depression and suggest consideration of screening for substance and alcohol dependence and/or abuse.[1] The Patient Health Questionnaire-2 (PHQ-2, **Box 4**) is a simple and rapid screening tool for depression, and patients screening positive for depression can be referred to their primary care physicians or specialists for further evaluation. The CAGE (cut back, angry, guilty, eye-opener) questionnaire can be used to screen for alcohol or substance dependence and abuse,[1] with a positive

---

Box 2
Cognitive assessment with the Mini-Cog: 3-item recall and clock draw

1. Get the patient's attention, then say:
   - "I am going to say 3 words that I want you to remember now and later. The words are: banana, sunrise, chair. Please say them for me now."
   - Give the patient 3 tries to repeat the words. If unable after 3 tries, go to the next item.

2. Say all the following phrases in the order indicated:
   - "Please draw a clock in the space below. Start by drawing a large circle. Put all the numbers in the circle and set the hands to show 11:10 (10 past 11)."
   - If the patient has not finished clock drawing in 3 minutes, discontinue and ask for recall items.

3. Say: "What were the 3 words I asked you to remember?"

From Chow WB, Rosenthal RA, Merkow RP, et al, American College of Surgeons National Surgical Quality Improvement Program, American Geriatrics Society. Optimal preoperative assessment of the geriatric surgical patient: a best practices guideline from the American College of Surgeons National Surgical Quality Improvement Program and the American Geriatrics Society. J Am Coll Surg 2012;215(4):455; with permission.

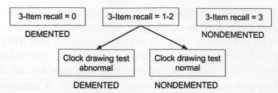

Fig. 1. Mini-Cog scoring algorithm. (*Adapted from* Borson S, Scanlan J, Brush M, et al. The Mini-Cog: a cognitive 'vital signs' measure for dementia screening in multi-lingual elderly. Int J Geriatr Psychiatry 2000;15(11):1024; with permission.)

response to any question considered a positive result. Patients who screen positive for alcohol or substance abuse are considered for perioperative withdrawal prophylaxis, referral for detoxification or abstinence programs, and perioperative multivitamin (including thiamine and folic acid) supplementation.

CARDIAC EVALUATION

Geriatric surgical patients, like all patients, should be evaluated from a cardiac standpoint according to the American College of Cardiology (ACC) and the American Heart Association (AHA) guidelines.[6] These guidelines were updated in 2014 to include an improved perioperative cardiac risk calculator that replaces the Revised Cardiac Risk Index. The new perioperative cardiac risk calculator is an interactive tool and quantifies risk based on the following 5 predictors: type of surgery, dependent functional status, abnormal creatinine level, American Society of Anesthesiologists (ASA) class, and increasing age.[7] It provides an exact probability for perioperative myocardial infarction or cardiac arrest (as opposed to stratification by high, intermediate, or low risk), which offers improved guidance when discussing informed consent and the risk/benefit profile of surgery.

PULMONARY EVALUATION

Postoperative pulmonary complications may include pneumonia and postoperative respiratory failure (PRF), defined as requiring mechanical ventilation greater than

Table 1
Legally relevant criteria for decision-making capacity and approaches to assessment of patients

Criteria	Patient's Task	Physician's Assessment Approach
Understanding	Grasp the fundamental meaning of information communicated by physician	Encourage patient to paraphrase information regarding medical condition and treatment
Appreciation	Acknowledge medical condition and likely consequences of treatment options	Ask patient to describe views of medical condition, proposed treatment, and likely outcomes
Reasoning	Engage in a rational discussion of the relevant information	Ask patient to compare treatment options and consequences and to offer reasons for selection of option
Choice	Indicate the preferred treatment option	Ask patient to indicate a treatment choice

Adapted from Appelbaum PS. Clinical practice. Assessment of patients' competence to consent to treatment. N Engl J Med 2007;357(18):1836.

Box 3
Risk factors for postoperative delirium

Cognitive and behavioral disorders

- Cognitive impairment
- Depression
- Alcohol use
- Sleep deprivation or disturbance

Disease or illness related

- Aortic procedures
- Current hip fracture
- Severe illness or comorbidity burden
- Presence of infection
- Renal insufficiency
- Inadequately controlled pain
- Anemia
- Hypoxia or hypercarbia

Metabolic

- Poor nutrition
- Dehydration
- Electrolyte abnormalities (hypernatremia or hyponatremia)

Functional impairments

- Hearing or vision impairment
- Poor functional status
- Immobilization or limited mobility

Other

- Age greater than 65 years
- Polypharmacy and use of psychotropic medications (benzodiazepines, anticholinergics, antihistamines, antipsychotics)
- Risk of urinary retention or constipation
- Presence of urinary catheter

Adapted from Chow WB, Rosenthal RA, Merkow RP, et al, American College of Surgeons National Surgical Quality Improvement Program, American Geriatrics Society. Optimal preoperative assessment of the geriatric surgical patient: a best practices guideline from the American College of Surgeons National Surgical Quality Improvement Program and the American Geriatrics Society. J Am Coll Surg 2012;215(4):453–66; and American Geriatrics Society Expert Panel on Postoperative Delirium in Older Adults. Postoperative delirium in older adults: best practice statement from the American Geriatrics Society. J Am Coll Surg 2015;220(2):136–48.e1.

48 hours after surgery or unplanned intubation within 30 days of surgery. Guidelines strongly recommend that geriatric patients are assessed for their risk of developing pulmonary complications preoperatively. A risk calculator was recently developed that, similar to the cardiac risk calculator, is an interactive tool that provides an exact probability for PRF based on 5 preoperative predictors: type of surgery, emergency

---

Box 4
The PHQ-2

1. In the past 12 months, have you ever had a time when you felt sad, blue, depressed, or down for most of the time for at least 2 weeks?

2. In the past 12 months, have you ever had a time, lasting at least 2 weeks, when you did not care about the things that you usually cared about or when you did not enjoy the things that you usually enjoyed?

If the patient answers "Yes" to either question, then further evaluation by a primary care physician or specialist is recommended.

From Chow WB, Rosenthal RA, Merkow RP, et al, American College of Surgeons National Surgical Quality Improvement Program, American Geriatrics Society. Optimal preoperative assessment of the geriatric surgical patient: a best practices guideline from the American College of Surgeons National Surgical Quality Improvement Program and the American Geriatrics Society. J Am Coll Surg 2012;215(4):455; with permission.

---

case, dependent functional status, preoperative sepsis, and higher ASA class.[8] Additional risk factors for postoperative pulmonary complications are detailed in **Box 5**. Preoperative strategies should be considered in order to reduce the risk of postoperative pulmonary complications, including medically optimizing patients with preexisting pulmonary disease, smoking cessation, preoperative intensive inspiratory muscle training, and selective chest radiograph and pulmonary function testing.[1]

FRAILTY

A critical perioperative measurement for geriatric patients is frailty. Frailty is defined as a decrease in physiologic reserve across multiple organ systems that renders the patient less able to deal with the physiologic stressors of surgery, anesthesia, and the postoperative period. In essence, the patient is less able to recover from perturbations in homeostasis.[9] The prevalence of frailty is higher in women and increases with age.[10] It is estimated that up to 50% of people more than 85 years of age may be frail.[11]

Frailty status, along with the patient's other comorbidities, predicts disability in the postoperative period; however, there is currently no standardized measure for frailty assessment.[11] An operational frailty score, developed by Fried and colleagues,[9] tabulates weight loss, grip strength, subjective low energy level, low physical activity, and slowness, to give a point tally defining degree of frailty. Additional definitions proposed by Robinson and colleagues[12] include cognitive impairment, poor nutrition, history of falls, low hematocrit, functional impairment, and comorbidity.

Sarcopenia and cachexia are other common characteristics associated with aging that are associated with poor quality of life and, ultimately, death.[11] Sarcopenia is suspected when the grip strength is in the lowest 20th percentile by gender and body mass index. Unintentional weight loss of more than 4.5 kg (10 pounds), or more than 10% of the person's body weight in the past year, should alert the anesthesiologist to the potential presence of cachexia. It is important for the anesthesiologist to recognize and document these two components as part of the frailty assessment to better characterize the overall clinical picture of the patient.[11]

Perioperative assessment of geriatric patients coming in for elective surgery should include some form of a measurement tool for frailty and, if time allows, an intervention to reduce their levels of frailty before surgery. At present, many interventional studies are underway to determine how best to do this, including vitamin and mineral

---

Box 5
Risk factors for postoperative pulmonary complications

Patient-related factors

- Age greater than 60 years
- Chronic obstructive pulmonary disease
- ASA class II or greater
- Functional dependence
- Congestive heart failure
- Obstructive sleep apnea
- Pulmonary hypertension
- Current cigarette use
- Impaired sensorium
- Preoperative sepsis
- Weight loss greater than 10% in 6 months
- Serum albumin level less than 3.5 mg/dL
- Blood urea nitrogen level greater than or equal to 7.5 mmol/L ($\geq$21 mg/dL)
- Serum creatinine level greater than 133 mol/L (>1.5 mg/dL)

Surgery-related factors

- Prolonged operation (>3 hours)
- Surgical site
- Emergency operation
- General anesthesia
- Perioperative transfusion
- Residual neuromuscular blockade after an operation

Adapted from Chow WB, Rosenthal RA, Merkow RP, et al, American College of Surgeons National Surgical Quality Improvement Program, American Geriatrics Society. Optimal preoperative assessment of the geriatric surgical patient: a best practices guideline from the American College of Surgeons National Surgical Quality Improvement Program and the American Geriatrics Society. J Am Coll Surg 2012;215(4):455; with permission.

---

supplementation, protein supplementation, exercise programs, the use of anabolic steroids and growth hormones, and angiotensin-converting enzyme inhibitors.[11]

Clinical evaluation for emergency surgery precludes optimization but still provides an opportunity to make a quick assessment of relative frailty and perhaps modify drug choices, and dosages, as well as determine postoperative disposition. Increased levels of frailty may alert anesthesiologists to pay closer attention to fluid status and other physiologic parameters in the perioperative period.[11]

FUNCTIONAL STATUS

Functional status assessment measures a patient's ability to perform activities of daily living and establishes a baseline in physical capacity. It has great prognostic ability for perioperative outcomes.[13] Furthermore, impaired functional status has been associated with poor postoperative outcomes.[14] A simple screening test to assess functional status consists of determining the patient's ability to get into and out of chairs unassisted, dress, bathe, prepare meals, and shop (eg, for groceries). If the patient is not able to perform any of these activities, a more in-depth screening needs to be performed and deficits documented. In addition, sensorineural deficits, such as vision or hearing, should be documented. Swallowing ability should also be noted, because this is important for postoperative nutrition. A history of falls should be documented, and gait and mobility testing should be performed using the Timed Up and Go Test (TUGT).[15] Any patient requiring more than 15 seconds to complete the test is at high risk of falls. Prolonged TUGT, and any functional dependence, have been found to be strong predictors for institutional rehabilitation postoperatively.[16]

NUTRITIONAL STATUS

Nutrition and nutritional status have important implications in the perioperative period, so a thorough evaluation of geriatric patients for nutritional deficiencies is a necessity. Preoperative evaluation should document height, weight, body mass index (BMI), serum albumin and prealbumin levels, and history of unintentional weight loss in the last 12 months. Patients are at severe nutritional risk if they have a BMI of less than 18.5 kg/m^2, serum albumin level less than 3.0 g/dL with no underlying cause such as renal or hepatic dysfunction, or more than 10% to 15% weight loss within the past 6 months.[1] If a patient is severely undernourished, a perioperative evaluation and plan by a dietician should be performed and implemented. If necessary, elective surgery may be postponed until better nutritional status is achieved, because poor nutritional status has been associated with increased risk of postoperative adverse events such as surgical site infections, pneumonia, urinary tract infections, and wound complications.[1]

MEDICATION HISTORY AND POLYPHARMACY

Because of limited reserve and increased sensitivity to medications and medication side effects, geriatric patients merit a tailored approach from a pharmacologic standpoint. Guidelines make the following recommendations:

1. Perform a comprehensive review and documentation of prescription and nonprescription medications.
2. Limit the prescription of new medications and consider discontinuing nonessential medications.
3. Identify medications that should be discontinued before surgery by consulting the updated Beers Criteria for potentially inappropriate medication use in older adults.[17]
4. Avoid starting new benzodiazepines and reduce benzodiazepines prescribed to patients at risk for delirium.
5. Avoid drugs such as meperidine for pain control and use caution when prescribing antihistamines or other medications with strong anticholinergic effects.[1]
6. Consider starting medications to decrease the perioperative risk of adverse cardiovascular events such as myocardial infarction and cardiovascular accident. Follow ACC/AHA guidelines for perioperative β-blockers and statins.[18]
7. Adjust doses of medications for renal function based on glomerular filtration rate, not on serum creatinine level alone.

DIAGNOSTIC TESTS

Geriatric surgical patients are a special subset of surgical patients who may require some baseline laboratory tests such as hemoglobin level/hematocrit, renal function tests, and albumin level. If the patient has had such laboratory tests within the past 4 months and has no marked change in clinical status, then prior laboratory results can safely be used. Diagnostic tests should only be performed if there is suspicion for the presence of disease based on symptoms or earlier testing. Testing may also be considered for higher-risk patients with known comorbidities, and/or those under-going higher-risk surgical procedures.[1]

PATIENT COUNSELING

It is highly recommended that geriatric patients have an advance directive and desig-nated health care proxy before arrival for elective surgery, and that copies of these documents are readily available. In addition, a review and documentation of the pa-tient's expectations, preferences, and goals for treatment is necessary to better improve communication between patients and their health care providers. This approach is good practice in general, but is especially important preoperatively because during the postoperative period the patient may not be in a position to communicate these things directly. Furthermore, it is important to determine family or friend support structures for the patient, and refer the patient to a social worker if the social support system is insufficient.[1]

FUTURE CONSIDERATIONS/SUMMARY

The preoperative assessment of geriatric patients is a multi–organ system challenge. Excellent screening and risk stratification tools exist for certain areas such as neuro-psychiatric, cardiac, pulmonary, and frailty evaluation. Future efforts need to be focused on widespread adoption of these guidelines as well as standardization of assessment tools.

REFERENCES

1. Chow WB, Rosenthal RA, Merkow RP, et al, American College of Surgeons Na-tional Surgical Quality Improvement Program, American Geriatrics Society. Optimal preoperative assessment of the geriatric surgical patient: a best prac-tices guideline from the American College of Surgeons National Surgical Quality Improvement Program and the American Geriatrics Society. J Am Coll Surg 2012; 215(4):453–66.
2. Nicholas JA. Preoperative optimization and risk assessment. Clin Geriatr Med 2014;30(2):207–18.
3. Borson S, Scanlan J, Brush M, et al. The Mini-Cog: a cognitive 'vital signs' mea-sure for dementia screening in multi-lingual elderly. Int J Geriatr Psychiatry 2000; 15(11):1021–7.
4. Appelbaum PS. Clinical practice. Assessment of patients' competence to con-sent to treatment. N Engl J Med 2007;357(18):1834–40.
5. American Geriatrics Society Expert Panel on Postoperative Delirium in Older Adults. Postoperative delirium in older adults: best practice statement from the American Geriatrics Society. J Am Coll Surg 2015;220(2):136–48.e1.
6. Fleisher LA, Fleischmann KE, Auerbach AD, et al. 2014 ACC/AHA guideline on perioperative cardiovascular evaluation and management of patients undergoing noncardiac surgery: a report of the American College of Cardiology/American Heart Association Task Force on Practice Guidelines. J Am Coll Cardiol 2014; 64(22):e77–137.

7. Gupta PK, Gupta H, Sundaram A, et al. Development and validation of a risk calculator for prediction of cardiac risk after surgery. Circulation 2011;124(4): 381–7.

8. Gupta H, Gupta PK, Fang X, et al. Development and validation of a risk calculator predicting postoperative respiratory failure. Chest 2011;140(5):1207–15.

9. Fried LP, Ferrucci L, Darer J, et al. Untangling the concepts of disability, frailty, and comorbidity: implications for improved targeting and care. J Gerontol A Biol Sci Med Sci 2004;59:255–63.

10. Amrock L, Deiner S. Geriatric anesthesia. In: Barnett SR, editor. Perioperative frailty. International anesthesiology clinics. Boston (MA): Lippincott Williams & Wilkins; 2014. p. 26–41.

11. Griffiths R, Mehta M. Frailty and anaesthesia: what we need to know. Cont Edu Anaesth Crit Care Pain 2014;14(6):273–7.

12. Robinson TN, Eiseman B, Wallace JI, et al. Redefining geriatric preoperative assessment using frailty, disability and comorbidity. Ann Surg 2009;250:449–55.

13. Hartmann SI, Barnett S. Geriatric anesthesia. In: Barnett SR, editor. Geriatric consultation. International anesthesiology clinics. Boston (MA): Lippincott Williams & Wilkins; 2014. p. 26–41.

14. Korc-Grodzicki B, Sung WS, Qin Z, et al. Geriatric assessment as a predictor of delirium and other outcomes in elderly patients with cancer. Ann Surg 2014;00: 1–6.

15. Summary of the Updated American Geriatrics Society/British Geriatrics Society clinical practice guideline for prevention of falls in older persons. J Am Geriatr Soc 2011;59:148–57.

16. Robinson TN, Wallace JI, Wu DS, et al. Accumulated frailty characteristics predict postoperative discharge institutionalization in the geriatric patient. J Am Coll Surg 2011;213:37–42 [discussion: 42–4].

17. American Geriatrics Society 2012 Beers Criteria Update Expert Panel. American Geriatrics Society updated Beers Criteria for potentially inappropriate medication use in older adults. J Am Geriatr Soc 2012;60:616–31.

18. Woolger JM. Preoperative testing and medication management. Clin Geriatr Med 2008;24:573–83, vii.

Optimal Preoperative Evaluation and Perioperative Care of the Geriatric Patient: A Surgeon's Perspective

CrossMark

Susan E. Wozniak, MD, MBA, JoAnn Coleman, DNP, ACNP-BC,
Mark R. Katlic, MD*

KEYWORDS

• Elderly • Geriatric • Frailty • Cognition • Preoperative • Screening

KEY POINTS

• The "Optimal Preoperative Assessment of the Geriatric Surgical Patient: A Best Practices Guideline," is a comprehensive assessment addressing domains most likely to affect the elderly: cognition, functionality, frailty, polypharmacy, nutrition, and social support.

• Even though a comprehensive "geriatric screening" may not be possible in a small clinical setting, options exist for a more limited geriatric preoperative assessment.

• Even when performing a more limited preoperative assessment, it will allow surgeons to improve surgical optimization and tailor planned procedures to individual patient needs.

• A geriatric preoperative assessment allows one to preemptively understand more clearly at what level to involve physical therapy, occupational therapy, social work, and other critical members of the operative care team.

INTRODUCTION

The aging of the population is rapidly changing the "landscape" of health care practice. This is particularly seen with the growth in numbers of the "oldest old," those older than 85 years. Surgeons encounter the "oldest old" on at least a monthly basis in their clinical practice. Conditions like atherosclerosis, cancer, degenerative joint disease, cataracts, and prostatism, common to the geriatric population, increase with increasing age.

Some centers have shown excellent results for surgery in the elderly, results equal to those in the general population. This even goes for complex operations

Department of Surgery, Sinai Center for Geriatric Surgery, Sinai Hospital, 2401 West Belvedere Avenue, Baltimore, MD 21215, USA
* Corresponding author.
E-mail address: mkatlic@lifebridgehealth.org

Anesthesiology Clin 33 (2015) 481–489
http://dx.doi.org/10.1016/j.anclin.2015.05.012   anesthesiology.theclinics.com

such as pancreaticoduodenectomy,[1–3] hepatectomy,[4–6] aortic arch replacement,[7] gastrectomy,[8,9] and esophagectomy[10–12] (**Fig. 1**). More importantly, it also has been shown that the quality of life in the elderly can be maintained or improved after surgery.[13–17]

Across the United States and around the world, age remains a risk factor for postoperative morbidity[18,19] and mortality.[20–23] Finlayson and colleagues[21] reported increased operative mortality in septuagenarians and octogenarians undergoing high-risk cancer operations (**Fig. 2**), a result mirrored in a study of 30,900 colorectal resections in the National Surgery Quality Improvement Program (NSQIP) database.[24] Aortoiliac aneurysm repair, whether open or endovascular, embodied increased risk of mortality for each 5 years older than 64 years in a recent study of 20,095 patients.[25] Postoperative length of stay is often longer than that in younger patients.[26,27] It bids the question as to how to match those centers that obtain excellent surgical results in the elderly? And, how can we all do better?

Improvement recommendations can be categorized into comprehensive preoperative evaluation and improved perioperative care. The former, the focus of this article, allows for more informed selection or denial of individual patients for surgery, encourages modifying the operation to each individual patient, and best informs the entire team caring for the individual patient. The repeated word "individual" is key, with decisions based on functional age rather than chronologic age.

A clear preoperative evaluation in the elderly, the Holy Grail of Geriatric Surgery,[28] is a simple, reliable test to assess perioperative risk. It must be fundamentally based on evidence and consensus, and if simple, it would be universally adopted in surgeons' offices and preoperative testing areas. This "Holy Grail" has not yet been found. Until then, we will continue establishing well-vetted best practice guidelines to optimize preoperative geriatric care.

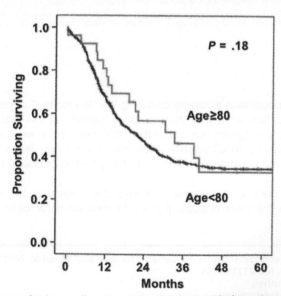

Fig. 1. Some centers obtain excellent operative results in elderly patients: pancreatectomy for cancer. (*From* Hatzaras I, Schmidt C, Klemanski D, et al. Pancreatic resection in the octogenarian: a safe option for pancreatic malignancy. J Am Coll Surg 2011;212(3):375; with permission.)

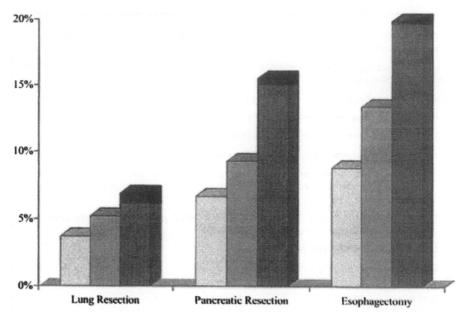

Fig. 2. In general, age is associated with increased perioperative risk: operative mortality of high-risk cancer operations in the United States by procedure and age. Light gray bar, aged 65 to 69 years; dark gray bar, aged 70 to 79 years; black bar, aged 80+ years. (*From* Finlayson E, Fan Z, Birkmeyer JD. Outcomes in octogenarians undergoing high-risk cancer operation: a national study. J Am Coll Surg 2007;205(6):730; with permission.)

THE AMERICAN COLLEGE OF SURGEONS/AMERICAN GERIATRICS SOCIETY BEST PRACTICE GUIDELINES

In 2012, the American College of Surgeons (ACS) NSQIP and the American Geriatrics Society (AGS) published "Optimal Preoperative Assessment of the Geriatric Surgical Patient: A Best Practice Guidelines."[29] Based on a focused, structured literature review, a 21-member multidisciplinary panel evaluated, over 4 rounds, a drafted set of recommendations and statements. The panel represented the 2 professional societies (ACS and AGS), the ACS Geriatric Surgery Task Force, 14 medical centers, and representatives of various surgical subspecialties, anesthesiology, and geriatric medicine. The preoperative domains addressed were those most likely to affect the elderly, including cognition, frailty, polypharmacy, nutrition, and social support.

Recognizing that this comprehensive evaluation (**Box 1**) would require time and resources, the panel nevertheless believed that those would be offset by the benefits of identifying high-risk individuals, improving communication between surgeon and patient, and potentially preventing adverse events. Is this evaluation really feasible, however, in a busy surgeon's office or busy preoperative assessment suite? Is a less extensive examination possible?

THE COMPLETE MEAL: BEST PRACTICES AND MORE

At the Sinai Center for Geriatric Surgery we have incorporated all of the ACS NSQIP/ AGS Best Practice Guidelines and have added several others: hearing screen, oral screen, performance status, Charlson Comorbidity Index, pressure ulcer risk, and caregiver burden interview. Our evaluation, performed by an experienced nurse

---

Box 1
ACS NSQIP/AGS best practices checklist for the optimal preoperative assessment of the geriatric surgical patient

In addition to conducting a complete and thorough history and physical examination of the patient, the following assessments are strongly recommended:

☐ Assess the patient's *cognitive ability* and *capacity* to understand the anticipated surgery.

☐ Screen the patient for *depression.*

☐ Identify the patient's risk factors for developing postoperative *delirium.*

☐ Screen for *alcohol* and other *substance abuse/dependence.*

☐ Perform a preoperative *cardiac* evaluation according to the American College of Cardiology/American Heart Association algorithm for patients undergoing noncardiac surgery.

☐ Identify the patient's risk factors for postoperative *pulmonary* complications and implement appropriate strategies for prevention.

☐ Document *functional status* and history of *falls.*

☐ Determine baseline *frailty* score.

☐ Assess the patient's *nutritional status* and consider preoperative interventions if the patient is at severe nutritional risk.

☐ Take an accurate and detailed *medication history* and consider appropriate perioperative adjustments. Monitor for *polypharmacy.*

☐ Determine the patient's *treatment goals* and *expectations* in the context of the possible treatment outcomes.

☐ Determine the patient's *family* and *social support system.*

☐ Order appropriate preoperative *diagnostic tests* focused on elderly patients.

Abbreviations: ACS, American College of Surgeons; AGS, American Geriatrics Society; NSQIP, National Surgical Quality Improvement Program.

From Chow WB, Rosenthal RA, Merkow RP, et al. Optimal preoperative assessment of the geriatric surgical patient: a best practices guideline from the American College of Surgeons National Surgical Quality Improvement Program and the American Geriatrics Society. J Am Coll Surg 2012;215(4):454; with permission.

---

practitioner on patients 75 years and older before any elective surgery, requires 20 to 30 minutes beyond a routine history and physical examination. It is carried out in our preoperative assessment area. Data are entered into a database within our Cerner electronic health record, accessible to all who care for the patient.

Problems identified preoperatively lead to more compulsive perioperative care. Alerts are placed in the chart for decreased hearing, fall risk, and pressure sore risk. Patients who fail the Mini-Cog test are targeted for measures to prevent postoperative delirium.[30] Our Social Service Department is notified if a patient's caregiver is found to be burdened preoperatively, as that patient is less likely to return directly home. Surgeons are called if their patient is frail, procedures are rarely canceled but operations may be modified, or if the patient does not demonstrate understanding of the planned procedure.

The financial commitment for this comprehensive program includes the salary and benefits of the nurse practitioner (who also contributes to the academic and educational mission of our center), a hand grip strength dynamometer (we use a Jamar; Sammons Preston Rolyan, Bolingbrook, IL), a screening audiometer (we use an

AudioScope; Welch Allyn, Skaneateles Falls, NY), information technology support to build the electronic database, and some printed material to educate our referring physicians. Patients potentially could be billed for a low-level evaluation to offset some of the expense. However, the chief benefits will be in decreased length of stay, fewer complications, and increased patient satisfaction; preliminary (Katlic MR, Coleman J, unpublished data, 2014) support this.

Is it necessary to do all of this, or would a more limited evaluation be possible? Are there other options that might be more practical in a different setting?

THE À LA CARTE MENU: MORE PRACTICAL OPTIONS FOR SOME

Options exist in a number of areas for a more practical approach to the geriatric preoperative evaluation: the person who performs the evaluation, the location of the evaluation, a more limited dataset of tests, the location of the data, and prospective versus retrospective study.

Who Performs the Evaluation

The clinical coordinator of our Center for Geriatric Surgery is a 30-year veteran of the department of surgery at a major university center, with a doctorate of nursing practice and a master's degree in adulthood and aging. However, she has taught others to do our complete evaluation, including residents and other nurse practitioners in the preoperative testing area. The total geriatric preoperative evaluation could be performed by a nurse, resident, medical student, physician assistant, or the patient's surgeon.

Location of the Evaluation

The preoperative testing area is ideal for the geriatric evaluation: many patients are there already for laboratory testing or a routine history and physical examination. However, any clinic or surgeon's office is suitable. The hand grip dynamometer and screening audiometer are portable (and potentially expendable, see later in this article) and timed-up-and-go, gait speed, Mini-Cog, and other tests can be completed anywhere. A hospital or department of surgery might decide to pilot the program in one specialty, one division, or one large surgery group.

Dataset of Tests

A more limited set of tests may prove to be 80% as good as our evaluation at 20% of the time commitment. A group of tests that cover the general domains of frailty, cognition, and function/performance status would add a great deal of information to the typical physical examination (**Table 1**).

The ACS NSQIP/AGS Best Practice Guidelines recommend a 5-point test of frailty popularized by Fried and colleagues[31] and proven valuable in a surgical population.[32,33] Others, however, have used simple gait speed[34] or the timed-up-and-go test.[35] A basic screen of cognition is the Mini-Cog test,[36] which involves a 3-item recall and clock-drawing; this simple test has been correlated with risk of worse postoperative results.[37] Activities of daily living (ADL), instrumental activities of daily living (IADL), and performance status (eg, Eastern Cooperative Oncology Group score) involve simple questions. Medication reconciliation and falls risk assessment have become routine already in many institutions.

Location of the Data

An electronic health record is optimal for the location of testing results, as it is accessible by all throughout the patient's perioperative course. If the database is

Table 1	
Comprehensive versus limited dataset of tests	
Comprehensive	**Limited (One from Each Domain)**
CAGE Screen for Alcohol Abuse	Cognition:
Cardiac and pulmonary risk factors	• Mini-Cog
Frailty, 5-point phenotype assessment	• MMSE
ADL	Frailty:
IADL	• 5-point
TUG	• Climbing
Nutrition screen	Function:
Hearing screen	• ECOG
Medication review	• ADL
Charlson Comorbidity Index score	• IADL
Advanced directive counseling	
Fall risk assessment	
Performance status, ECOG	
Stair-climbing question	
Living situation	
Quality of life/health rating	
Estimated creatinine clearance/GFR	
Postoperative delirium risk factors	
Caregiver burden interview	
Provider "Gestalt" assessment	
Oral/dental screen	
Pincher strength assessment	

Abbreviations: ADL, activities of daily living; CAGE, cut-down, annoyed, guilty, eye-opener; ECOG, Eastern Cooperative Oncology Group Performance Scale; GFR, glomerular filtration rate; IADL, instrumental activities of daily living; MMSE, Mini Mental Status Examination; TUG, timed up-and-go test.

constructed with discrete fields, it may be queried subsequently for research or quality improvement purposes. A paper form that follows the patient is also possible, as is a simple addendum to the dictated history and physical examination.

Allowing access to the geriatric assessment allows not only the surgical management team but also physical therapy, occupational therapy, nursing, and social workers to understand more clearly the patient's baseline. Physical and occupational therapy are able to better gauge a patient's preoperative activity status, as physician admission notes often do not contain important information regarding details covered in a geriatric preoperative assessment. Social workers can often anticipate in advance what additional services they may need to obtain for the patient before discharge.

Prospective or Retrospective

Everything that has been presented in this article is meant to be done prospectively, as the patient is being evaluated preoperatively for surgical fitness. Hospitals that participate in ACS NSQIP may have the option in the future of abstracting geriatric variables 30 days or more after the patient's operation. These new variables, being piloted in 22 hospitals in 2014, include preoperative cognitive status and use of mobility aid, postoperative pressure ulcer, delirium, ADLs, and more.

SUMMARY

The elderly preoperative patient benefits from an assessment that includes more than a routine physical examination and electrocardiogram. Such an assessment includes domains likely to affect the elderly: cognition, functionality, frailty, polypharmacy, nutrition, and social support. This fosters decisions based on functional age rather than chronologic age and on each patient as an individual.

One such assessment is that promulgated by the ACS NSQIP/AGS Best Practice Guidelines. If this comprehensive evaluation is considered impractical for an institution or surgeon's office, a limited dataset of tests will still be valuable. We should not miss any opportunity to improve results in this growing population of surgical patients.

REFERENCES

1. Petrowsky H, Clavien PA. Should we deny surgery for malignant hepato-pancreatico-biliary tumors to elderly patients? World J Surg 2005;29(9): 1093–100.
2. Hatzaras I, Schmidt C, Klemanski D, et al. Pancreatic resection in the octogenarian: a safe option for pancreatic malignancy. J Am Coll Surg 2011;212(3):373–7.
3. Buchs NC, Addeo P, Bianco FM, et al. Outcomes of robot-assisted pancreatico-duodenectomy in patients older than 70 years: a comparative study. World J Surg 2010;34(9):2109–14.
4. Ferrero A, Vigano L, Polastri R, et al. Hepatectomy as treatment of choice for hepatocellular carcinoma in elderly cirrhotic patients. World J Surg 2005;29(9): 1101–5.
5. Menon KV, Al-Mukhtar A, Aldouri A, et al. Outcomes after major hepatectomy in elderly patients. J Am Coll Surg 2006;203(5):677–83.
6. Kondo K, Chijiiwa K, Funagayama M, et al. Hepatic resection is justified for elderly patients with hepatocellular carcinoma. World J Surg 2008;32(10):2223–9.
7. Shah PJ, Estrera AL, Miller CC 3rd, et al. Analysis of ascending and transverse aortic arch repair in octogenarians. Ann Thorac Surg 2008;86(3):774–9.
8. Kunisaki C, Akiyama H, Nomura M, et al. Comparison of surgical outcomes of gastric cancer in elderly and middle-aged patients. Am J Surg 2006;191(2): 216–24.
9. Biondi A, Cananzi FC, Persiani R, et al. The road to curative surgery in gastric cancer treatment: a different path in the elderly? J Am Coll Surg 2012;215(6): 858–67.
10. Internullo E, Moons J, Nafteux P, et al. Outcome after esophagectomy for cancer of the esophagus and GEJ in patients aged over 75 years. Eur J Cardiothorac Surg 2008;33(6):1096–104.
11. Rice DC, Correa AM, Vaporciyan AA, et al. Preoperative chemoradiotherapy prior to esophagectomy in elderly patients is not associated with increased morbidity. Ann Thorac Surg 2005;79(2):391–7 [discussion: 391–7].
12. Ruol A, Portale G, Zaninotto G, et al. Results of esophagectomy for esophageal cancer in elderly patients: age has little influence on outcome and survival. J Thorac Cardiovasc Surg 2007;133(5):1186–92.
13. Amemiya T, Oda K, Ando M, et al. Activities of daily living and quality of life of elderly patients after elective surgery for gastric and colorectal cancers. Ann Surg 2007;246(2):222–8.
14. Hamel MB, Toth M, Legedza A, et al. Joint replacement surgery in elderly patients with severe osteoarthritis of the hip or knee: decision making, postoperative recovery, and clinical outcomes. Arch Intern Med 2008;168(13):1430–40.
15. Zierer A, Melby SJ, Lubahn JG, et al. Elective surgery for thoracic aortic aneurysms: late functional status and quality of life. Ann Thorac Surg 2006;82(2): 573–8.

16. Huber CH, Goeber V, Berdat P, et al. Benefits of cardiac surgery in octogenarians–a postoperative quality of life assessment. Eur J Cardiothorac Surg 2007; 31(6):1099–105.
17. Moller A, Sartipy U. Changes in quality of life after lung surgery in old and young patients: are they similar? World J Surg 2010;34(4):684–91.
18. Ngaage DL, Cowen ME, Griffin S, et al. Early neurological complications after coronary artery bypass grafting and valve surgery in octogenarians. Eur J Cardiothorac Surg 2008;33(4):653–9.
19. Leo F, Scanagatta P, Baglio P, et al. The risk of pneumonectomy over the age of 70. A case-control study. Eur J Cardiothorac Surg 2007;31(5):780–2.
20. Turrentine FE, Wang H, Simpson VB, et al. Surgical risk factors, morbidity, and mortality in elderly patients. J Am Coll Surg 2006;203(6):865–77.
21. Finlayson E, Fan Z, Birkmeyer JD. Outcomes in octogenarians undergoing high-risk cancer operation: a national study. J Am Coll Surg 2007;205(6):729–34.
22. Moskovitz AH, Rizk NP, Venkatraman E, et al. Mortality increases for octogenarians undergoing esophagogastrectomy for esophageal cancer. Ann Thorac Surg 2006;82(6):2031–6 [discussion: 2036].
23. Seeburger J, Falk V, Garbade J, et al. Mitral valve surgical procedures in the elderly. Ann Thorac Surg 2012;94(6):1999–2003.
24. Kiran RP, Attaluri V, Hammel J, et al. A novel nomogram accurately quantifies the risk of mortality in elderly patients undergoing colorectal surgery. Ann Surg 2013; 257(5):905–8.
25. Tsilimparis N, Perez S, Dayama A, et al. Age-stratified results from 20,095 aortoiliac aneurysm repairs: should we approach octogenarians and nonagenarians differently? J Am Coll Surg 2012;215(5):690–701.
26. Barnett SD, Halpin LS, Speir AM, et al. Postoperative complications among octogenarians after cardiovascular surgery. Ann Thorac Surg 2003;76(3):726–31.
27. Jarvinen O, Huhtala H, Laurikka J, et al. Higher age predicts adverse outcome and readmission after coronary artery bypass grafting. World J Surg 2003; 27(12):1317–22.
28. Katlic MR. The Holy Grail of geriatric surgery. Ann Surg 2013;257(6):1005–6.
29. Chow WB, Rosenthal RA, Merkow RP, et al. Optimal preoperative assessment of the geriatric surgical patient: a best practices guideline from the American College of Surgeons National Surgical Quality Improvement Program and the American Geriatrics Society. J Am Coll Surg 2012;215(4):453–66.
30. Inouye SK, Bogardus ST Jr, Charpentier PA, et al. A multicomponent intervention to prevent delirium in hospitalized older patients. N Engl J Med 1999;340(9): 669–76.
31. Fried LP, Tangen CM, Walston J, et al. Frailty in older adults: evidence for a phenotype. J Gerontol A Biol Sci Med Sci 2001;56(3):M146–56.
32. Revenig LM, Canter DJ, Taylor MD, et al. Too frail for surgery? Initial results of a large multidisciplinary prospective study examining preoperative variables predictive of poor surgical outcomes. J Am Coll Surg 2013;217(4):665–70.e1.
33. Makary MA, Segev DL, Pronovost PJ, et al. Frailty as a predictor of surgical outcomes in older patients. J Am Coll Surg 2010;210(6):901–8.
34. Afilalo J, Eisenberg MJ, Morin JF, et al. Gait speed as an incremental predictor of mortality and major morbidity in elderly patients undergoing cardiac surgery. J Am Coll Cardiol 2010;56(20):1668–76.
35. Robinson TN, Wu DS, Sauaia A, et al. Slower walking speed forecasts increased postoperative morbidity and 1-year mortality across surgical specialties. Ann Surg 2013;258(4):582–8 [discussion: 588–90].

36. Borson S, Scanlan J, Brush M, et al. The mini-cog: a cognitive 'vital signs' measure for dementia screening in multi-lingual elderly. Int J Geriatr Psychiatry 2000; 15(11):1021–7.
37. Robinson TN, Wu DS, Pointer LF, et al. Preoperative cognitive dysfunction is related to adverse postoperative outcomes in the elderly. J Am Coll Surg 2012; 215(1):12–7 [discussion: 17–8].

Anesthetic Considerations for Common Procedures in Geriatric Patients

Hip Fracture, Emergency General Surgery, and Transcatheter Aortic Valve Replacement

Laeben Lester, MD

KEYWORDS

- Geriatric anesthesia • Elderly anesthesia • Anesthesia emergency surgery
- Anesthesia TAVR • Hip fracture • Emergency general surgery
- Transcatheter aortic valve replacement

KEY POINTS

- Focused history and physical before going to the operating room is essential, even in patients with extensive preoperative evaluation given risk for changing condition.
- Pay special attention to pharmacokinetic and neurologic differences associated with aging.
- Consider regional anesthesia with light sedation for geriatric patients undergoing surgery for hip fracture.
- Emergency abdominal surgery is very high risk and requires coordinated and timely supportive care.
- Transcatheter aortic valve replacement is an emerging treatment for aortic stenosis that will proliferate rapidly.

INTRODUCTION

The elderly population is growing, and citizens 65 and over will increase from 13% of the population in 2010 to 20% by 2030.[1] Geriatric patients undergo a large proportion of operative procedures and have increased complications, morbidity, and mortality, which may be associated with increased intensive care unit (ICU) time, length of stay, hospital readmission, and high cost.[2,3] With the expanding elderly population,

Division of Cardiothoracic Anesthesia, Department of Anesthesiology and Critical Care Medicine, Johns Hopkins School of Medicine, 1800 Orleans Street, Zayed 6208, Baltimore, MD 21287-7294, USA
E-mail address: llester4@jhmi.edu

Anesthesiology Clin 33 (2015) 491–503
http://dx.doi.org/10.1016/j.anclin.2015.05.006
1932-2275/15/$ – see front matter © 2015 Elsevier Inc. All rights reserved.
anesthesiology.theclinics.com

identification of optimal anesthetic care for the older patient that leads to decreased complications and contributes to the best possible outcomes will have outsized value for individual patients and society.

This article reviews the anesthetic considerations for intraoperative care of geriatric patients and focuses on 3 procedures that are common, high risk, and/or emerging. First, an approach to evaluation and management of the elderly surgical patient is described. Then, a review of anesthetic management for repair of hip fractures, emergency abdominal surgery, and transcatheter aortic valve replacement (TAVR) are discussed.

GENERAL APPROACH TO ANESTHETIC MANAGEMENT IN THE ELDERLY PATIENT

Advancing age, American Society of Anesthesiologists status, low preoperative albumin concentration, and frailty are all risk factors for perioperative complications and mortality.[2,4] Complications are associated with increased morbidity and mortality, and neurologic, cardiovascular, respiratory, renal, and infectious complications are common.[2,4,5] Anesthetic management should be tailored to prevent and adequately manage perioperative complications while maintaining appropriate surgical conditions, patient safety and patient comfort.[6,7] A high level of postoperative care is necessary in the high-risk elderly patient, and ICU admission should be considered for prompt recognition and management of complications.[8] General anesthesia, regional anesthesia, and local anesthesia with sedation, as well as combined general and regional or local anesthesia, can all be performed safely in elderly patients. Overall, there is no specific anesthetic technique that has proved superior to others.[9–11] However, in the case of hip fracture, this balance seems to be tipping in favor of regional anesthesia; this issue is discussed elsewhere in this article.[12,13]

Focused History and Physical

Preoperative evaluation and optimization of the elderly patient over 65 is essential[14] and are discussed in detail in the article by Tsai and Nakhaie elsewhere in this issue. A focused history and physical evaluating for new or underappreciated conditions is prudent, even after prior preoperative evaluation and optimization.

Consider Pharmacologic Differences

The pharmacologic differences between older and younger patients are complex, involve both pharmacokinetic and pharmacodynamics interactions, and are discussed in depth in articles by Akhtar and Ramani, elsewhere in this issue.[15] In practice, these changes lead to increased sensitivity to anesthetic agents and decreased dose requirements.[15] Impatience and lack of appreciation of delayed time to peak effect and increased sensitivity associated with aging can lead to "dose stacking"—a dangerous overshooting of the desired effect. To avoid dose stacking, slow, gentle titration of intravenous anesthetics such as propofol, with a dose that may be 50% of the weight-based dose in younger adults, is necessary. Hypotension should be anticipated and treated.[16]

Consider the Systems-Based Changes Associated with Aging

The physiologic differences associated with aging are discussed in depth elsewhere in this issue. A brief mental review of physiologic changes associated with airway, breathing, circulation, disability (neurologic), renal and electrolyte, hepatic, endocrine, hematologic, and infectious disease is helpful in avoiding pitfalls.

Routine precautions and best practices for any major surgery should also be provided vigilantly for geriatric patients, including timely and appropriate antibiotic treatment and deep vein thrombosis prophylaxis. Careful positioning of the frail, elderly patient may be particularly important because they may be at increased risk of spinal stenosis, decubitus ulcer, and tearing of the skin. Particular attention to maintenance of normothermia in the frail, elderly patient is also important, because hypothermia has been associated with increased risk of myocardial ischemia.[17]

ANESTHETIC CONSIDERATIONS FOR HIP FRACTURES

Fragility fractures—hip fractures in elderly patients from low-impact falls associated with osteoporosis—are the second most common reason for hospital admission in elderly patients.[18,19] Hip fractures account for significant morbidity, mortality, and cost.[20,21] Surgery of the hip, femur, and knee are among the most commonly performed operative procedures in patients 65 years and older and the percent contribution to overall surgeries increases with age. In patients greater than 90 years of age, treatment of hip and femur fractures and dislocations accounted for 22.2% and partial or total hip replacement an additional 4.9% of surgeries performed at hospitals reporting to the National Anesthesia Clinical Outcomes Registry.[22,23] Surgery for hip fractures and hip replacement are associated with a high risk of perioperative complications in elderly patients, increasing costs, and decreasing value.[20,23]

Immediate Preoperative Considerations

In general, the patient with a hip fracture presents to the emergency department for evaluation and stabilization before proceeding to the inpatient ward or operating room. A focused history, physical, and review of prior evaluations is prudent before going to the operating room, especially if the cause of the fall is not established. Delay in time to operation is a risk factor for poor perioperative outcomes in the geriatric patient and has been associated with worse outcomes, increased duration of stay, and decubitus ulcers.[24,25] Therefore, it is important to minimize delay to surgery for patients who are optimized for the operating room.[19]

General Versus Regional Anesthesia

Although it remains controversial, the majority of studies comparing regional versus general anesthesia suggest that regional anesthesia may be superior.[12,26–29] In 2012, Neuman and colleagues[12] retrospectively analyzed the records of more than 18,000 patients undergoing surgery for hip fracture and found regional anesthesia associated with a 25% to 29% decrease in major pulmonary events and mortality, with this potential difference attributed to intratrochanteric fractures rather than femoral neck fractures. Memtsoudis and colleagues[28] evaluated data from 382,236 records and showed a decreased major morbidity and mortality rate associated with regional anesthesia for patients undergoing total knee arthroplasty and a trend toward lesser major morbidity and mortality for total hip arthroplasty. In 2014, Neuman and colleagues[26] evaluated 56,729 records of patients undergoing surgery for hip fracture and found no difference in mortality, but a decreased duration of stay. However, other studies have suggested longer duration of stay or increased complications with regional anesthesia compared with general anesthesia,[23,30] and earlier Cochrane reviews have suggested no difference between general and regional anesthesia for hip fractures.[31]

Regional anesthesia is usually administered with sedation, but few studies comparing general anesthesia and regional anesthesia have focused on depth of anesthesia and sedation. Recently, Sieber and colleagues[32] conducted a randomized trial of light sedation (Bispectral Index of ~50) versus deep sedation (Bispectral Index pf >80) in older adults undergoing hip fracture repair under spinal anesthesia. They found a 50% reduction in the incidence of delirium in the light sedation group. In a follow-up survival analysis, Brown and colleagues[13] found that, in patients with serious comorbidities, mortality was significantly reduced at 1 year in the light sedation group. These findings suggest that, in the highest risk elderly patients, regional anesthesia with light sedation may be superior to regional anesthesia with deep sedation, although further research is needed.

Pharmacologic Considerations

Patients with hip long bone fracture are at high risk for deep vein thrombosis and prophylaxis should be initiated preoperatively and continued through the intraoperative and postoperative course to prevent deep vein thrombosis and pulmonary embolus; pressure gradient stockings should be worn.[33] Prevention of pressure ulcers can begin in the perioperative period and can reduce morbidity significantly and improve outcomes.[19]

Increasingly, goals of care after fixation of hip fracture are early mobilization and rehabilitation. Rapid recovery from anesthesia and sedation while maintaining adequate pain control is important, and can be obtained with patient-controlled analgesia or patient-controlled epidural analgesia.[19]

ANESTHETIC CONSIDERATIONS FOR EMERGENT GENERAL SURGERY

Emergent gastrointestinal surgery is associated with high morbidity and mortality rates, especially in elderly patients.[34] The 30-day mortality rates for patients over the age of 80 undergoing emergency laparotomy are reported from 24% to 44%.[35,36] Morbidity and mortality seem to increase with emergency surgery and age.[37] The proportion of surgeries that are urgent and emergent also seems to increase with age.[22] More than 40% of patients presenting for emergency general surgery present with systemic inflammatory response syndrome, sepsis, or septic shock.[38] Delay in surgery seems to be associated with worse outcomes, especially in patients with sepsis.[39] Postoperative admission to the ICU may be associated with fewer complications and better outcomes in high-risk patients, including elderly patients.[8,40]

Immediate Preoperative Considerations

Patients presenting for urgent and emergent surgery require rapid history, physical examination, evaluation of laboratory analysis, and review of diagnostic tests. In particular, early abdominal imaging is important to aid in diagnosis and guide surgical management.[41] The patient with ongoing hemorrhage requires immediate surgery.[42] Evaluation for systemic inflammatory response syndrome, sepsis, and septic shock are essential given the high prevalence in patients presenting for emergent gastrointestinal surgery.[38] Early antibiotic administration with broad-spectrum antibiotics is required because the duration of hypotension before antibiotic administration is a critical determinant of survival in septic shock.[43] Initiation of goal-directed resuscitation with restoration of euvolemia, subsequent vasopressor support with norepinephrine for vasodilation, and optimization of oxygen delivery is indicated.[44] Once the decision to proceed to surgery is made, the patient should go to the operating room as soon as possible.

The emergency laparotomy pathway quality improvement care (ELPQuiC) bundle was recently implemented in 4 hospitals in the United Kingdom and showed a significant reduction in the risk of death after emergency laparotomy[41] (**Table 1**).

Intraoperative Considerations

General anesthesia is indicated for patients requiring emergent gastrointestinal surgery given the emergent nature of the case, the open abdomen, and the high likelihood of hemodynamic instability and need for ongoing resuscitation.[39] The use of combined general and epidural anesthesia may be indicated in some patients. However, the risk of hypotension and infection in the patient with sepsis and/or ongoing bleeding may outweigh the benefits of postoperative pain control that may be associated with epidural anesthesia. Further, routine precautions as outlined elsewhere in this article should be followed, with particular focus on temperature management in the elderly patient undergoing emergent gastrointestinal surgery.

Pharmacologic Considerations

Patience with hypovolemia and shock will have altered hepatic and renal blood flow and function, which may contribute to prolonged and unpredictable effects of anesthetic agents. Likewise, the hemodynamic effects of anesthetic agents may be pronounced. Ketamine and etomidate are generally considered to be the most hemodynamically stable agents for induction of anesthesia in the patient with hypovolemia or shock[45] Maintenance anesthetic may need to be decreased, which may increase the risk of awareness. Continued anesthetic management, including adjunctive ketamine, midazolam, and scopolamine, may be necessary. However, administration of benzodiazepine and scopolamine in the geriatric patient may increase the risk of delirium.

Airway

Patients presenting for emergent gastrointestinal surgery are at high risk for aspiration.[46] The goals of intraoperative management are to safely and quickly secure the airway while minimizing the risk of aspiration without worsening shock. Rapid sequence intubation or modified rapid sequence intubation is most commonly used to facilitate intubation and minimize the risk of active regurgitation.

Table 1
The 5 elements of the ELPQuiC bundle

	ELPQuiC Bundle
1.	Early assessment with early warning scoring on presentation with graded escalation policies for senior clinical evaluation and ICU referral
2.	Broad-spectrum antibiotics to all patients with fecal soiling or any evidence of sepsis
3.	Once decision is made to go to surgery, the patient takes the next available operating room (or within 6 h of the decision being made)
4.	Start resuscitation using goal-directed techniques as soon as possible, or within 6 h of admission
5.	Admit all patients to the ICU after emergency laparotomy

Abbreviations: ELPQuiC, emergency laparotomy pathway quality improvement care bundle; ICU, intensive care unit.

Data from Huddart S, Peden CJ, Swart M, et al. Use of a pathway quality improvement care bundle to reduce mortality after emergency laparotomy. Br J Surg 2015;102(1):57–66.

Breathing
Low tidal volume ventilation with tidal volumes of 5 to 8 mL/kg have been advocated as a lung protective strategy, and this may be particularly important in the elderly emergent gastrointestinal surgery patient who may be at increased risk for acute respiratory distress syndrome.[44] The patient in shock with fever may have increased myocardial oxygen demand, which may further increase the risk of desaturation with the induction of apnea for intubation.

Circulation
The patient with distributive shock is at significant risk for hypotension with induction of anesthesia and the initiation of positive-pressure ventilation, and may require placement of an arterial line before the induction of anesthesia. Likewise, a fluid bolus before induction may be prudent. If not already started, initiation of anesthetic vasopressor medications, particularly norepinephrine, may be indicated before or immediately after induction if they have not been started previously. Arterial pressure monitoring is necessary during emergent gastrointestinal surgery in the elderly patient.[45] Central access for medication administration and monitoring of the central venous pressure may also be required, and allow estimation of central venous SVO_2.[44] Additional monitoring with arterial waveform analysis for cardiac output or pulmonary artery catheter may be necessary in some patients. Likewise, transesophageal echocardiography may be helpful if severe hypotension is unresponsive to fluid, pressor, and inotropic administration.

Renal and electrolyte
Maintenance of renal perfusion is a goal of resuscitation. Maintenance of urine output is reassuring, but may be abnormal in the geriatric patient taking diuretics or other medications. Electrolyte abnormalities should be followed. Acidosis, particularly gap acidosis, is suggestive of shock and the need for continued resuscitation. In the setting of hypotension, severe acidosis can be treated with sodium bicarbonate.

Hepatic
Coagulopathy may be associated with hemodilution, hemorrhage, sepsis or hepatic dysfunction owing to shock.

Endocrine
Severe hyperglycemia should be controlled with intravenous insulin. Although it may be rare, hypotension that is not responsive to fluid and pressor medications can be owing to adrenal insufficiency. Likewise, induction with a single dose of etomidate causes measurable decreases in cortisol that is of unknown significance in clinical practice.

Positioning
Care in positioning the patient should be taken because elderly patients may be at increased risk for decubitus ulcers.

Postoperative Period
Elderly patients undergoing emergent gastrointestinal surgery are considered high risk and generally are admitted to the ICU for ongoing resuscitation.[41] Patients requiring ventilator support, ongoing hemodynamic instability, or resuscitation, or those with persistent acidosis should continue with ongoing ventilatory support and delayed extubation in the ICU.

ANESTHETIC CONSIDERATIONS FOR TRANSCATHETER AORTIC VALVE REPLACEMENT

TAVR is emerging as a less invasive treatment for severe aortic stenosis than surgical aortic valve replacement. At the heart of the TAVR procedure is the deployment of an expandable, prosthetic valve in the aortic valve position. TAVR is most commonly performed with retrograde delivery through the transfemoral approach, and this approach is the focus of this discussion. Additional approaches include subclavian, axillary, direct aortic, and apical delivery.[47] A transcaval approach involving placement through the IVC into the abdominal aorta has also been described.[48]

The emergence of TAVR is particularly relevant to the anesthetic care of geriatric patients. Degenerative aortic stenosis is the most common valvular heart disease in Western countries and the prevalence increases with age.[49] In patients greater than 65 years old, the prevalence is 2%, and in patients older than 80 years it is more than 4%.[49,50] In symptomatic patients—those with angina, syncope, or heart failure—the mortality rate is very high, approximately 50% in the first 2 years.[51] Medical management in severe aortic stenosis is not particularly effective, and many frail, elderly patients with comorbidities are high risk for surgical aortic valve replacement and some are extreme risk or inoperable.[52,53] TAVR has emerged as an option for patients with inoperable or extreme risk, and as an alternative to surgery for high-risk patients.[53,54] TAVR procedures are being performed with increasing frequency, and are performed primarily on high-risk elderly patients. Therefore, TAVR is an important emerging procedure in the geriatric population. Ongoing trials of TAVR for intermediate risk surgical patients could further expand the role of this new intervention in the elderly patient population.[47]

Two devices currently have approval from the Food and Drug Administration (FDA) in the United—the Edward Sapien Transcatheter Heart Valve (THV; Edward Life Sciences Inc, Irvine, CA) and the Medtronic CoreValve System (Medtronic Inc, Minneapolis, MN). The Edward Sapien THV is a balloon expandable bioprosthetic aortic valve on a steel scaffold. The first multicenter, randomized, controlled trial Placement of AoRTic TransCathetER Valve (PARTNER) showed a survival advantage with TAVR in inoperable patients compared with medical therapy or balloon valvuloplasty, and a second cohort comparing TAVR with surgical aortic valve replacement (SAVR) in high-risk patients showed noninferiority, with no difference in 30-day and 1-year all-cause mortality.[53] These findings led to FDA approval for the Edward Sapien THV in 2011 and 2012 for patients at extreme surgical risk or who were considered inoperable, and as an alternative to SAVR in high-risk candidates, respectively. An updated version, the Edwards Sapien XT THV with a cobalt chromium tubular alloy frame, more sizing options, and updated delivery system, was approved in 2014. The Medtronic CoreValve System is a bioprosthetic valve supported by a self-expanding nitinol frame. The US CoreValve Investigators' randomized, controlled trials showed a survival advantage with TAVR over medical therapy in patients at prohibitive risk for SAVR, and a 1-year survival advantage compared with SAVR in high-risk surgical patients.[54,55] These findings in turn led to stepwise FDA approval for patients at extreme or prohibitive surgical risk in January of 2014 and for high-risk candidates in June 2014.

TAVR procedures are usually performed in a hybrid cardiovascular suite with fluoroscopic equipment and the ability to perform cardiothoracic surgery with cardiopulmonary bypass available. During the procedure, vascular access is often performed percutaneously, but may require cutdown to the femoral artery. Both femoral arteries are accessed, with a pigtail catheter placed in the opposite artery for administration of contrast dye. Placement of a right ventricular pacemaker is confirmed to allow rapid placement during procedure (at our institution, this is placed by anesthesia through a 6-Fr cordis, usually in the right internal jugular vein). The femoral artery is dilated, the introducer sheath is positioned carefully, and the wire is placed retrograde across the aortic valve. The valve is deployed, usually under rapid pacing (not always necessary with CoreValve). Positioning and valve function are evaluated by fluoroscopy and transesophageal or transthoracic echocardiography.

Complications can be catastrophic and include vascular injury, hemorrhage, pericardial bleeding and tamponade, conduction abnormalities and arrhythmias, myocardial ischemia and infarction, valve malpositioning, stroke, and renal injury.[53–56]

Patient Selection

TAVR is indicated for patients with severe, symptomatic aortic stenosis who are at high or prohibitive risk for SAVR. High risk is based on a Society for Thoracic Surgery risk score of greater than 10% or Logistic EuroSCORE of greater than 20%[47]; of these, the Society for Thoracic Surgery risk score is likely more representative of high-risk SAVR.[57] Current recommendations from the American College of Cardiology/American Heart Association Valvular Heart Disease Guidelines recommend surgical aortic valve replacement if the predicted risk of mortality is less than 8%, and TAVR for frail, elderly patients with comorbidities placing them at more significant risk for SAVR. A multidisciplinary team evaluation is advocated, including cardiologists, cardiothoracic surgeons, and anesthesiologists.[58]

Immediate Preoperative Considerations

TAVR patients typically undergo extensive preoperative evaluation and are most often optimized for the procedure. Given the high-risk, elderly population with severe aortic stenosis and multiple comorbidities, a focused history and physical examination is necessary before going to the procedure suite. Particular attention should be paid to development of new or worsening cardiac symptoms, including chest pain, dyspnea, syncope, dependent edema, palpitations, and orthopnea.

Anesthetic Management: General Anesthesia Versus Procedural Sedation

Both general anesthesia and monitored anesthesia care (MAC) with sedation and adjunctive local anesthetic are used in the anesthetic management of patients undergoing transfemoral TAVR.[47] General anesthesia is more commonly used in North America, and MAC is more common in Europe.[59] One retrospective study recently compared device success and cumulative 30-day survival in 2326 patients undergoing TAVR with general anesthesia versus MAC and showed no difference in device success and cumulative 30 day survival, but did show a higher rate of post-TAVR aortic regurgitation greater than mild in the sedation group that may have been owing to increased use of transesophageal echocardiography in the GA group.[60] MAC may be a safe option, but emergency conversion to general anesthesia has been reported to be as high as 17%, mainly owing to complications of the procedure, including hemorrhage, cardiac tamponade, cardiac arrest, myocardial ischemia, and stroke.[59,61]

At our institution, we perform TAVR under both general anesthesia and MAC. When general anesthesia is performed, induction is performed after placement of an awake arterial line and anesthesia is maintained with desflurane 3% to 4% and low-dose fentanyl (≤100 μg for the entire case), and preoperative oral or intraoperative intravenous acetaminophen is often administered. Transesophageal echocardiography is performed routinely when general anesthesia is used, and is especially valuable for evaluation of the valve after deployment. A 6-Fr introducer sheath is usually placed in the right internal jugular vein through which a transvenous pacemaker is placed, and later floated into the right ventricle under fluoroscopy. In patients who have no risk factors for difficult airway, can lie flat without difficulty, have no pulmonary hypertension, uncomplicated vascular anatomy, and no other risk factors for difficult TAVR, MAC with sedation and local anesthesia is performed.

Airway
TAVR is usually an elective procedure in optimized patients with severe aortic stenosis. A slow, controlled induction after an arterial line is placed is followed by endotracheal intubation. Patients with risk factors for difficult intubation can be extubated awake and are generally not candidates for MAC given the potential need to rapidly control the airway if complications with the procedure arise.

Breathing
Patients with severe aortic stenosis are at risk for hypotension and ischemia with positive-pressure ventilation and decreased left ventricular preload. They are also at risk for pulmonary edema with volume overload.

Circulation
TAVR patients have severe aortic stenosis. Maintenance of coronary perfusion pressure is critical. This requires maintenance of preload, afterload, and maintenance of left ventricular filling with a low normal heart rate. Phenylephrine is often useful for hypotension. Hemodynamic monitoring with an arterial pressure line is required. Central venous access with pacing is usually necessary to allow for overdrive pacing to decrease the cardiac output during balloon angiography and deployment of the Edwards Sapien valve. Recovery after pacing can be slow and may require vasopressor or inotropic support. Arrhythmias during wire manipulation or valve deployment can cause hypotension and cardiac arrest. Ischemia owing to calcium emboli or occlusion of the coronary os can be catastrophic.

Disability

Renal
Renal perfusion pressure and euvolemia should be maintained given the significant contrast load and increased risk of renal injury.

Endocrine
Diabetes is common in this population and extreme glucose should be treated.

Positioning and skin
Patients receive a clopidogrel loading dose (600 mg) and may be on anticoagulants. Gentle padding and taping are required. Special care should be taken to avoid injury to lips with transesophageal echocardiography probe.

FUTURE DIRECTIONS

Ongoing research is needed to establish best practices for anesthetic management of elderly patients undergoing surgical procedures. This includes determining if regional anesthesia with light sedation produces better outcomes than general anesthesia in hip fractures, improving coordinated care for geriatric patients undergoing emergent gastrointestinal surgery, and establishing optimal anesthetic management for the emerging TAVR procedure. TAVR represents an emerging therapy for elderly patients with severe degenerative aortic stenosis and is likely to proliferate rapidly.

REFERENCES

1. Vincent GK, Velkoff VA. The next four decades, the older population in the United States: 2010–2050, current population reports, current population reports. Current Population Reports. Washington, DC: US Census Bureau; 2010. p. P25–1138.
2. Hamel MB, Henderson WG, Khuri SF, et al. Surgical outcomes for patients aged 80 and older: morbidity and mortality from major noncardiac surgery. J Am Geriatr Soc 2005;53(3):424–9.
3. Polanczyk CA, Marcantonio E, Goldman L, et al. Impact of age on perioperative complications and length of stay in patients undergoing noncardiac surgery. Ann Intern Med 2001;134(8):637–43.
4. McNicol L, Story DA, Leslie K, et al. Postoperative complications and mortality in older patients having non-cardiac surgery at three Melbourne teaching hospitals. Med J Aust 2007;186(9):447–52.
5. Jin F, Chung F. Minimizing perioperative adverse events in the elderly. Br J Anaesth 2001;87(4):608–24.
6. Story DA. Postoperative complications in elderly patients and their significance for long-term prognosis. Curr Opin Anaesthesiol 2008;21(3):375–9.
7. Sieber FE, Barnett SR. Preventing postoperative complications in the elderly. Anesthesiol Clin 2011;29(1):83–97.
8. Vester-Andersen M, Lundstrom LH, Moller MH, et al. Mortality and postoperative care pathways after emergency gastrointestinal surgery in 2904 patients: a population-based cohort study. Br J Anaesth 2014;112(5):860–70.
9. Christopherson R, Beattie C, Frank SM, et al. Perioperative morbidity in patients randomized to epidural or general anesthesia for lower extremity vascular surgery. Perioperative Ischemia Randomized Anesthesia Trial Study Group. Anesthesiology 1993;79(3):422–34.
10. Dodds TM, Burns AK, DeRoo DB, et al. Effects of anesthetic technique on myocardial wall motion abnormalities during abdominal aortic surgery. J Cardiothorac Vasc Anesth 1997;11(2):129–36.
11. Liu SS, Strodtbeck WM, Richman JM, et al. A comparison of regional versus general anesthesia for ambulatory anesthesia: a meta-analysis of randomized controlled trials. Anesth Analg 2005;101(6):1634–42.
12. Neuman MD, Silber JH, Elkassabany NM, et al. Comparative effectiveness of regional versus general anesthesia for hip fracture surgery in adults. Anesthesiology 2012;117(1):72–92.
13. Brown CH 4th, Azman AS, Gottschalk A, et al. Sedation depth during spinal anesthesia and survival in elderly patients undergoing hip fracture repair. Anesth Analg 2014;118(5):977–80.
14. McGory ML, Kao KK, Shekelle PG, et al. Developing quality indicators for elderly surgical patients. Ann Surg 2009;250(2):338–47.
15. Vuyk J. Pharmacodynamics in the elderly. Best Pract Res Clin Anaesthesiol 2003; 17(2):207–18.
16. Dundee JW, Robinson FP, McCollum JS, et al. Sensitivity to propofol in the elderly. Anaesthesia 1986;41(5):482–5.
17. Frank SM, Beattie C, Christopherson R, et al. Unintentional hypothermia is associated with postoperative myocardial ischemia. The perioperative ischemia randomized anesthesia trial study group. Anesthesiology 1993; 78(3):468–76.
18. Wilkins CH, Birge SJ. Prevention of osteoporotic fractures in the elderly. Am J Med 2005;118(11):1190–5.

19. Beaupre LA, Jones CA, Saunders LD, et al. Best practices for elderly hip fracture patients. A systematic overview of the evidence. J Gen Intern Med 2005;20(11): 1019–25.
20. Braithwaite RS, Col NF, Wong JB. Estimating hip fracture morbidity, mortality and costs. J Am Geriatr Soc 2003;51(3):364–70.
21. Cheng SY, Levy AR, Lefaivre KA, et al. Geographic trends in incidence of hip fractures: a comprehensive literature review. Osteoporos Int 2011;22(10):2575–86.
22. Deiner S, Westlake B, Dutton RP. Patterns of surgical care and complications in elderly adults. J Am Geriatr Soc 2014;62(5):829–35.
23. Basques BA, Bohl DD, Golinvaux NS, et al. Postoperative length of stay and 30-day readmission after geriatric hip fracture: an analysis of 8434 patients. J Orthop Trauma 2015;29(3):e115–20.
24. Henderson CY, Ryan JP. Predicting mortality following hip fracture: an analysis of comorbidities and complications. Ir J Med Sci 2015. [Epub ahead of print].
25. Ryan DJ, Yoshihara H, Yoneoka D, et al. Delay in hip fracture surgery: an analysis of patient- and hospital-specific risk factors. J Orthop Trauma 2015. [Epub ahead of print].
26. Neuman MD, Rosenbaum PR, Ludwig JM, et al. Anesthesia technique, mortality, and length of stay after hip fracture surgery. JAMA 2014;311(24):2508–17.
27. Luger TJ, Kammerlander C, Luger MF, et al. Mode of anesthesia, mortality and outcome in geriatric patients. Z Gerontol Geriatr 2014;47(2):110–24.
28. Memtsoudis SG, Sun X, Chiu YL, et al. Perioperative comparative effectiveness of anesthetic technique in orthopedic patients. Anesthesiology 2013;118(5): 1046–58.
29. Patorno E, Neuman MD, Schneeweiss S, et al. Comparative safety of anesthetic type for hip fracture surgery in adults: retrospective cohort study. BMJ 2014;348: g4022.
30. Whiting PS, Molina CS, Greenberg SE, et al. Regional anaesthesia for hip fracture surgery is associated with significantly more perioperative complications compared with general anaesthesia. Int Orthop 2015. [Epub ahead of print].
31. Parker MJ, Handoll HH, Griffiths R. Anaesthesia for hip fracture surgery in adults. Cochrane Database Syst Rev 2004;(4):CD000521.
32. Sieber FE, Zakriya KJ, Gottschalk A, et al. Sedation depth during spinal anesthesia and the development of postoperative delirium in elderly patients undergoing hip fracture repair. Mayo Clin Proc 2010;85(1):18–26.
33. Mak JC, Cameron ID, March LM. National Health and Medical Research Council. Evidence-based guidelines for the management of hip fractures in older persons: an update. Med J Aust 2010;192(1):37–41.
34. Griner D, Adams A, Kotwall CA, et al. After-hours urgent and emergent surgery in the elderly: outcomes and prognostic factors. Am Surg 2011;77(8):1021–4.
35. Cook TM, Day CJ. Hospital mortality after urgent and emergency laparotomy in patients aged 65 yr and over. Risk and prediction of risk using multiple logistic regression analysis. Br J Anaesth 1998;80(6):776–81.
36. Saunders DI, Murray D, Pichel AC, et al. UK Emergency Laparotomy Network. Variations in mortality after emergency laparotomy: the first report of the UK emergency laparotomy network. Br J Anaesth 2012;109(3):368–75.
37. Louis DJ, Hsu A, Brand MI, et al. Morbidity and mortality in octogenarians and older undergoing major intestinal surgery. Dis Colon Rectum 2009;52(1):59–63.
38. Ingraham AM, Cohen ME, Raval MV, et al. Comparison of hospital performance in emergency versus elective general surgery operations at 198 hospitals. J Am Coll Surg 2011;212(1):20–8.e1.

39. Peden C, Scott MJ. Anesthesia for emergency abdominal surgery. Anesthesiol Clin 2015;33(1):209–21.
40. Khuri SF, Henderson WG, DePalma RG, et al. Determinants of long-term survival after major surgery and the adverse effect of postoperative complications. Ann Surg 2005;242(3):326–41 [discussion: 341–3].
41. Huddart S, Peden CJ, Swart M, et al. Use of a pathway quality improvement care bundle to reduce mortality after emergency laparotomy. Br J Surg 2015;102(1): 57–66.
42. Stoneham M, Murray D, Foss N. Emergency surgery: the big three–abdominal aortic aneurysm, laparotomy and hip fracture. Anaesthesia 2014;69(Suppl 1):70–80.
43. Kumar A, Roberts D, Wood KE, et al. Duration of hypotension before initiation of effective antimicrobial therapy is the critical determinant of survival in human septic shock. Crit Care Med 2006;34(6):1589–96.
44. Dellinger RP, Levy MM, Rhodes A, et al. Surviving sepsis campaign: international guidelines for management of severe sepsis and septic shock: 2012. Crit Care Med 2013;41(2):580–637.
45. Gray LD, Morris C. The principles and conduct of anaesthesia for emergency surgery. Anaesthesia 2013;68(Suppl 1):14–29.
46. Orlando Hung MM, editor. Management of the difficult and failed airway. 1st edition. New York: McGraw-Hill; 2008.
47. Klein AA, Skubas NJ, Ender J. Controversies and complications in the perioperative management of transcatheter aortic valve replacement. Anesth Analg 2014; 119(4):784–98.
48. Greenbaum AB, O'Neill WW, Paone G, et al. Caval-aortic access to allow transcatheter aortic valve replacement in otherwise ineligible patients: initial human experience. J Am Coll Cardiol 2014;63(25 Pt A):2795–804.
49. Stewart BF, Siscovick D, Lind BK, et al. Clinical factors associated with calcific aortic valve disease. Cardiovascular Health Study. J Am Coll Cardiol 1997; 29(3):630–4.
50. Iung B, Baron G, Butchart EG, et al. A prospective survey of patients with valvular heart disease in Europe: the Euro Heart Survey on Valvular Heart Disease. Eur Heart J 2003;24(13):1231–43.
51. Otto CM. Timing of aortic valve surgery. Heart 2000;84(2):211–8.
52. Iung B, Cachier A, Baron G, et al. Decision-making in elderly patients with severe aortic stenosis: why are so many denied surgery? Eur Heart J 2005;26(24): 2714–20.
53. Leon MB, Smith CR, Mack M, et al. Transcatheter aortic-valve implantation for aortic stenosis in patients who cannot undergo surgery. N Engl J Med 2010; 363(17):1597–607.
54. Adams DH, Popma JJ, Reardon MJ, et al. Transcatheter aortic-valve replacement with a self-expanding prosthesis. N Engl J Med 2014;370(19):1790–8.
55. Popma JJ, Adams DH, Reardon MJ, et al. Transcatheter aortic valve replacement using a self-expanding bioprosthesis in patients with severe aortic stenosis at extreme risk for surgery. J Am Coll Cardiol 2014;63(19):1972–81.
56. Smith CR, Leon MB, Mack MJ, et al. Transcatheter versus surgical aortic-valve replacement in high-risk patients. N Engl J Med 2011;364(23):2187–98.
57. Wendt D, Thielmann M, Kahlert P, et al. Comparison between different risk scoring algorithms on isolated conventional or transcatheter aortic valve replacement. Ann Thorac Surg 2014;97(3):796–802.
58. Nishimura RA, Otto CM, Bonow RO, et al. 2014 AHA/ACC guideline for the management of patients with valvular heart disease: a report of the American College

of Cardiology/American Heart Association Task Force on Practice Guidelines. J Thorac Cardiovasc Surg 2014;148(1):e1–132.

59. Bufton KA, Augoustides JG, Cobey FC. Anesthesia for transfemoral aortic valve replacement in North America and Europe. J Cardiothorac Vasc Anesth 2013; 27(1):46–9.

60. Oguri A, Yamamoto M, Mouillet G, et al. Clinical outcomes and safety of transfemoral aortic valve implantation under general versus local anesthesia: subanalysis of the French Aortic National CoreValve and Edwards 2 registry. Circ Cardiovasc Interv 2014;7(4):602–10.

61. Bergmann L, Kahlert P, Eggebrecht H, et al. Transfemoral aortic valve implantation under sedation and monitored anaesthetic care–a feasibility study. Anaesthesia 2011;66(11):977–82.

Postoperative Delirium in the Geriatric Patient

Katie J. Schenning, MD, MPH[a],*, Stacie G. Deiner, MD[b,c,d]

KEYWORDS

- Postoperative delirium • Geriatric • Risk factors • Screening • Management

KEY POINTS

- Delirium is a common postoperative complication in the geriatric population.
- Postoperative delirium is independently associated with increased morbidity and mortality.
- Validated screening tools are useful for early detection.
- Treatment is aimed at addressing underlying causes and managing symptoms.

INTRODUCTION

Postoperative delirium (POD) is a common complication in older surgical patients and is associated with significantly prolonged hospitalizations, cognitive impairment, functional decline, and increased 6- to 12-month mortality rate.[1–5] Postoperative delirium has a reported incidence from 10% to 70% depending on the criteria used for diagnosis, the population studied, and the type of surgical procedure. Higher incidences tend to be reported in the oldest, most medically complex patients after vascular, cardiac, or hip fracture operations.[6–9] Skills essential for clinicians involved in the perioperative care of geriatric patients include the ability to (1) identify high-risk patients, (2) promptly diagnose POD, and (3) effectively manage patients with POD.

Funding sources: K12 HD 043488 and Oregon Alzheimer's Disease Center P30AG008017 (Dr K.J. Schenning). NIA R01- 13-0359-01001-01-PD7 (Dr S.G. Deiner).
Conflicts of Interest: None.
[a] Department of Anesthesiology & Perioperative Medicine, Oregon Health & Science University, 3181 SW Sam Jackson Park Road, Mail Code: HRC 5N, Portland, OR 97239, USA; [b] Department of Anesthesiology, Icahn School of Medicine at Mount Sinai, 1 Gustave L. Levy Place, Box 1010, New York, NY 10029, USA; [c] Department of Neurosurgery, Icahn School of Medicine at Mount Sinai, 1 Gustave L. Levy Place, Box 1010, New York, NY 10029, USA; [d] Department of Geriatrics and Palliative Care, Icahn School of Medicine at Mount Sinai, 1 Gustave L. Levy Place, Box 1010, New York, NY 10029, USA
* Corresponding author.
E-mail address: malcore@ohsu.edu

RISK FACTORS

Postoperative delirium is a complex, geriatric syndrome that results from interplay between a patient's baseline vulnerabilities (predisposing factors) and the insults that occur throughout the perioperative course (precipitating factors; **Table 1**).[10] Although many of the predisposing risk factors are not amenable to change, identification of patients with these factors can allow caregivers to direct preventive efforts to at-risk patients (see Management below). Because of the heterogeneity of the populations studied, research methodologies, and the syndrome itself, the reported risk factors for postoperative delirium vary. Predisposing risk factors frequently cited include age older than 65 years, functional impairment, preexisting neuropsychiatric conditions, and the presence of multiple medical comorbidities. Specific comorbidities associated with the development of postoperative delirium include heart failure, renal dysfunction, diabetes mellitus, and vascular disease.[11]

Together with knowledge of the predisposing factors, an understanding of the precipitating factors to which patients are exposed in the perioperative period can assist in directing perioperative care tailored to the individual patient. Although there is little evidence implicating a particular anesthetic agent or technique, emerging evidence suggests that the depth of anesthesia might play a role (see Current Controversies below). Other factors related to an increased risk of postoperative delirium include increased surgical duration, complexity, and invasiveness. Postoperative factors implicated in the development of delirium include admission to an intensive care unit, prolonged intubation/mechanical ventilation, poor pain management, and disrupted sleep patterns.

DIAGNOSIS

Delirium is an acute confusional state with symptoms that wax and wane throughout the course of the illness. Because delirium is a complex syndrome with a variable

---

Table 1
Risk factors for postoperative delirium

Predisposing Factors	Precipitating Factors
Age (>65 y)	Intraoperative
Neuropsychiatric conditions	• Blood loss/blood transfusion
• Cognitive dysfunction	• Surgery duration
• Dementia	• Surgical urgency
• Depression	• Surgical complexity
• Alcohol abuse	• Invasiveness of procedure
• History of postoperative delirium	• Depth of anesthesia
• History of stroke	Postoperative
Use of psychotropic medications	• Admission to an ICU
Poor physical status	• Increased hospital/ICU length of stay
Medical comorbidities	• Increased duration of intubation/mechanical
• Heart failure	ventilation
• Kidney failure	• Postoperative complications
• Diabetes mellitus	○ Infection, stroke
• Atrial fibrillation	• Use of physical restraints
• Anemia	• Sleep disruption
• Atherosclerosis	• Pain
• Tobacco use	• Psychotropic medication use

Abbreviation: ICU, intensive care unit.

clinical picture, clinicians must maintain a high index of suspicion to promptly detect postoperative delirium. Considering that delirium represents an acute or subacute change from baseline, it is important that each patient's baseline cognitive status is well documented.[12,13] The diagnosis of delirium is based on history, physical examination, and laboratory and radiographic findings. Other neurocognitive disorders should be ruled out to confirm the diagnosis of delirium (**Box 1**).

Clinical Features

On average, the onset of delirium begins 24 hours postoperatively and resolves within 48 hours.[14] Delirium, as defined in the Diagnostic and Statistical Manual of Mental Disorders (DSM), Fifth Edition, is a disturbance in attention, awareness, and cognition that develops over a short period and fluctuates in severity.[15] Clinically, delirium can take the form of hyperactive, hypoactive, or a mixed type that includes both hyperactive and hypoactive symptoms. Of these forms, the hypoactive subtype may be associated with the worst prognosis.[16,17] Other symptoms associated with delirium are listed in **Box 2**.

Screening Tools

Several validated tools are used for the screening and diagnosis of delirium (**Table 2**). Several of these screening instruments, including the Confusion Assessment Method (CAM)[18] and the Delirium Symptom Interview,[19] were developed using criteria adapted from the DSM. Routine screening of at-risk patients using a validated screening tool facilitates early diagnosis, particularly in the hypoactive form of delirium, which might otherwise go unrecognized. Despite the recent advances in validated tools, none of them is foolproof. It can be particularly challenging to diagnose delirium in patients with preexisting cognitive impairment, dementia, or psychiatric conditions.

PATHOPHYSIOLOGY

The pathophysiology of postoperative delirium is not entirely known; however, many theories exist regarding the underlying processes behind the clinical syndrome. As described by Maldonado[24] in his landmark review, potential mechanisms can be grouped into categories including neuroinflammation and oxidative stress. These 2 areas likely interact to cause delirium by promoting neurotransmitter dysregulation and network disconnectivity causing an imbalance in the activation or inhibition of neural networks (in specific cholinergic and GABAergic systems).[25,26] Below we describe the neuroinflammation and oxidative stress hypotheses in brief, as these areas span a large amount of literature.

Box 1
Differential diagnosis of postoperative delirium
Emergence delirium
Postoperative cognitive dysfunction
Cerebrovascular accident/transient ischemic attack
Dementia
Depression or other psychiatric conditions

> **Box 2**
> **Clinical features of postoperative delirium**
>
> Disturbance in attention, awareness, cognition, memory, concentration
>
> Fluctuating severity of symptoms
>
> Emotional lability
>
> Agitation
>
> Hallucinations or delusions
>
> Disorganized thoughts or speech
>
> Difficulty tracking conversations
>
> Change in sleep-wake cycle
>
> Change in level of arousal
>
> Decreased appetite
>
> Urinary/bowel incontinence
>
> Change in activity level
>
> • Hyperactive
>
> • Hypoactive
>
> • Mixed

Neuroinflammation

The peripheral neuroendocrine response to the stress of surgery and anesthesia leads to neuroinflammation. The immune and inflammatory response to stress activates the hypothalamic-pituitary-adrenal axis and induces the production of glucocorticoids. Glucocorticoids have a wide range of peripheral and central effects including the enhancement of neuroinflammation and ischemic injury.[27] The peripheral neuroendocrine response is propagated centrally via either the neural pathway (vagus nerve) activated by the hypothalamic-pituitary-adrenal axis or the humoral pathway by peripheral mediators crossing the blood-brain barrier. With respect to the humoral pathway, there is some evidence that peripheral mediators impact the brain at the choroid plexus and circumventricular organs leading to the production of proinflammatory cytokines in the brain.[28] Studies have explored peripheral inflammatory markers for delirium including C-reactive protein, tumor necrosis factor, and interleukin (IL)-6, IL-8, and IL-10.[29–31] Although these markers are found to be significantly elevated in patients with delirium, they are not specific for delirium.[32,33]

Neuroinflammation produces a syndrome of physiologic and behavioral changes termed *sickness behaviors*, which are not specific to the postoperative period, and are common for many systemic illnesses.[34] Sickness behaviors, which are thought to be part of the adaptive response to injury, include depression, cognitive deficits, and social withdrawal. According to this theory, delirium is considered an exaggerated form of a sickness behavior.

Oxidative Stress

The oxidative stress hypothesis proposes that brain hypoperfusion induces local ischemia, which triggers a chain of events. First, there is an increased production of reactive oxygen species. The increase in reactive oxygen species leads to

Table 2			
Validated delirium screening instruments			
Tool	**Sensitivity (%)**	**Specificity (%)**	**Criteria**
CAM[18]	94–100	90–95	9 criteria from DSM-III-R: acute onset and fluctuating course, inattention, disorganized thinking, altered level of consciousness, disorientation, memory impairment, perceptual disturbances, increased or decreased psychomotor activity, sleep-wake cycle disturbance
CAM for the Intensive Care Unit (CAM-ICU)[20]	95–100	89–93	4 items: acute onset or fluctuating course, inattention, disorganized thinking, altered level of consciousness
Delirium Symptom Interview[19]	90	80	7 criteria from DSM-III: disorientation, consciousness, sleep-wake cycle, perceptual disturbance, speech, psychomotor activity, fluctuating behavior
Nursing Delirium Screening Scale[21]	85.7	86.8	5 items: disorientation, behavior, communication, hallucinations, psychomotor retardation
Intensive Care Delirium Screening Checklist[22]	99	64	8 items: altered level of consciousness, inattention, disorientation, psychosis, psychomotor agitation/retardation, inappropriate speech/mood, sleep/wake cycle, symptom fluctuation
Neelon and Champagne Confusion Scale[23]	95	78	9 items in the following 3 domains: processing, behavior, physiologic control

excitotoxicity, apoptosis, and local inflammation. Because of melatonin's properties as a free radical scavenger, an antioxidant, and a regulator of circadian rhythm, its use in delirium prevention was explored.[35] However, a recent randomized, double-blind study of the administration of tryptophan, a precursor to melatonin, in older surgical patients found no difference in the incidence or duration of delirium.[36] Overall, the clinical evidence supporting the theory that global cerebral desaturation is a common cause of delirium is poor. A recent study compared the rate of postoperative delirium in patients undergoing cardiopulmonary bypass graft procedures with the Haga Brain Care Strategy with historical controls who did not receive the protocol. The Haga Brain Care Strategy included preoperative transcranial Doppler examinations and intraoperative cerebral oximetry. Cerebral desaturations that were greater than 20% outside of the normal range resulted in intervention to restore oxygenation. The study found that patients who underwent surgery with the protocol had a 7.3% incidence of delirium versus a 13.3% incidence in the historical control, which was statistically significant.[37] However, because patients undergoing general surgery rarely experience severe cerebral desaturation, this strategy may not be widely generalizable.[38] One small study of geriatric abdominal surgery patients suggested that patients who had delirium had lower preoperative regional oxygen saturation.[39] Overall, the cardiac and noncardiac studies that examined cerebral oximetry were small, retrospective, or a post hoc comparison of a parent study with a different endpoint. In the future, stronger evidence is needed to define whether cerebral hypoxia is a common cause of delirium in older surgery patients.

MANAGEMENT

Prevention, screening, and early treatment are the mainstays of postoperative delirium management. Most preventive strategies are nonpharmacologic as outlined in **Box 3**. In one randomized trial, a proactive geriatrics consultation reduced the incidence of postoperative delirium by more than one-third after hip fracture repair.[40] In this program, structured geriatrics consultations made recommendations regarding supplemental oxygen, fluids, electrolytes, nutrition, pain management, and early mobilization and physical rehabilitation. In an early landmark study, Inouye and colleagues[41] used a multicomponent intervention that decreased the incidence of delirium by 40% and the duration of delirium by 35%.[41] This strategy, which became known as the Hospital Elder Life Program, was directed toward managing the following 6 issues: cognitive impairment, sleep deprivation, immobility, visual impairment, hearing impairment, and dehydration. Although most strategies for delirium prevention are nonpharmacologic, the prophylactic use of ketamine or antipsychotics has shown some early success. These studies are further described under Current Controversies below.

After making the diagnosis of delirium, health care providers should attempt to identify and correct the underlying causes (**Box 4**). The use of pharmacologic strategies in managing postoperative delirium has a role in the treatment of the underlying medical causes and management of symptoms. For example, medications are particularly helpful in addressing underlying causes of delirium such as pain[42] or sleep deprivation. The American Geriatrics Society released a delirium best practices statement this fall.[12] The panel spent a year performing a Cochrane-style review to identify rigorously performed studies of factors to prevent and treat delirium. According to these

---

Box 3
Strategies for postoperative delirium prevention

Orient to setting

Increase mobility, physical therapy

Promote sleep hygiene

Proactive geriatrics consultation

Multicomponent interventions (ie, Hospital Elder Life Program)

Appropriate medication management

- Control pain
- Avoid polypharmacy
- Decrease use of medications with psychoactive properties

Ensure access to glasses, contacts, hearing aids, dentures

Educate health care personnel

Box 4
Potential underlying causes of delirium
Infection
Sleep deprivation
Inadequate pain control
Sedating/psychoactive medications
Metabolic/electrolyte derangements
Alcohol/drug intoxication or withdrawal

guidelines, the use of antipsychotics should be reserved for patients who are severely agitated and pose a risk to harm themselves or others.[12]

CURRENT CONTROVERSIES AND FUTURE CONSIDERATIONS

In the Delirium Best Practices Statement, the American Geriatrics Society panel found that the only intraoperative intervention that had the quality of evidence required to make a recommendation for clinical care was anesthetic depth.[12] This does not mean that other intraoperative factors (drugs, hemodynamics, cerebral saturation) have no effect on delirium but that more high-quality studies are needed.

Based on a pilot study of depth of anesthesia in geriatric hip fracture patients, the Best Practices Statement suggests that anesthesiologists should avoid deep planes of anesthesia to prevent delirium. The guideline does mention that the risks of light anesthesia are not insignificant, and these include intraoperative awareness and sympathetic system activation.[12] Further evidence supporting this recommendation comes from a study of depth of sedation in patients who underwent hip fracture surgery under spinal anesthesia.[43] This finding was consistent with those of 2 larger trials in which the rate of postoperative delirium was lower in patients who received intraoperative Bispectral Index (BIS, Covidien, Boulder, CO, USA) monitoring versus patients who did not.[44,45] However, these 2 trials did not assign or randomly select patients to a particular depth of anesthesia. A study that randomly assigned hip fracture patients to light or heavy sedation is currently underway.

Use of Ketamine

A small randomized trial of a single bolus dose of ketamine or saline placebo after induction (0.5 mg/kg) showed impressive results. Patients who received ketamine had a 3% incidence of delirium compared with 31% of patients who received placebo.[46] The patients who received ketamine also had a significantly lower C-reactive protein level; therefore, the authors postulated that ketamine might have a salutary anti-inflammatory effect. Other mechanisms by which ketamine could attenuate the oxidative stress associated with surgery include inhibition of N-methyl-D-aspartate receptor activation and excitotoxic signaling and reduction of neural apoptosis.[47] Currently, a multicenter trial called Prevention of Delirium and Complications Associated with Surgical Treatments (PODCAST) is underway to study the effects of a bolus dose of ketamine in a noncardiac surgical population on postoperative delirium and pain.[48]

Use of Antipsychotics

The Best Practices Guidelines found insufficient evidence to recommend the use of antipsychotics to prevent delirium based the current contradictory literature and

> **Box 5**
> **Candidate biomarkers for postoperative delirium**
>
> Inflammatory (Interleukins, microglial activity, C-reactive protein, erythrocyte sedimentation rate, human leukocyte antigen–DR, CD68)
>
> Dopamine receptors
>
> Noradrenergic (Norepinephrine, cortisol)
>
> Cerebral damage (S-100β, neuron-specific enolase)
>
> Genetic (apolipoprotein E ε4)
>
> Cholinergic (acetylcholinesterase)
>
> Albumin levels

considerable harm of antipsychotics.[12,49–53] Currently there is an ongoing Dutch multicenter trial (Haloperidol Prophylaxis in Older Emergency Department Patients, HARPOON study) to determine efficacy and safety of haloperidol prophylaxis in at-risk patients.[54] Medical and surgical patients identified as high risk for delirium in the emergency department will be randomly assigned to 1 mg haloperidol prophylaxis twice daily for 7 days with delirium incidence as the primary endpoint and secondary endpoints including delirium free days, length of stay, and mortality. Regarding the use of antipsychotics for the purpose of treating delirium, the current guidelines recommend the lowest effective dose for the shortest duration and only after nonpharmacologic interventions have failed.

Potential Biomarkers

As mentioned, postoperative delirium is a complex syndrome associated with varied phenotypes and is likely the result of a combination of neuroinflammatory and oxidative stress processes. As such, biomarker investigations have generally focused on inflammatory, noradrenergic, ischemic, and anticholinergic markers[55] (**Box 5**). For example, postoperative norepinephrine levels were recently found to be much higher in postoperative patients in whom delirium developed.[56] Few studies have explored the genetic factors that predispose patients to postoperative delirium. Although some have found the presence of the apolipoprotein E ε4 allele increases the risk of postoperative delirium,[57,58] other studies found no association between the apolipoprotein E ε4 allele and delirium.[59]

SUMMARY

Postoperative delirium is a common complication plaguing geriatric surgical patients and is independently associated with increased morbidity and mortality. Successful management of postoperative delirium requires an understanding of which patients are at the highest risk for postoperative delirium development and a proactive approach to diagnosis and treatment.

REFERENCES

1. Dubljanin-Raspopovic E, Markovic Denic L, Marinkovic J, et al. Use of early indicators in rehabilitation process to predict one-year mortality in elderly hip fracture patients. Hip Int 2012;22(6):661–7.

2. Bickel H, Gradinger R, Kochs E, et al. High risk of cognitive and functional decline after postoperative delirium. A three-year prospective study. Dement Geriatr Cogn Disord 2008;26(1):26–31.
3. Kat MG, Vreeswijk R, de Jonghe JF, et al. Long-term cognitive outcome of delirium in elderly hip surgery patients. A prospective matched controlled study over two and a half years. Dement Geriatr Cogn Disord 2008;26(1):1–8.
4. Zakriya K, Sieber FE, Christmas C, et al. Brief postoperative delirium in hip fracture patients affects functional outcome at three months. Anesth Analg 2004; 98(6):1798–802. Table of contents.
5. Saczynski JS, Marcantonio ER, Quach L, et al. Cognitive trajectories after postoperative delirium. N Engl J Med 2012;367(1):30–9.
6. Parikh SS, Chung F. Postoperative delirium in the elderly. Anesth Analg 1995; 80(6):1223–32.
7. van der Mast RC, Roest FH. Delirium after cardiac surgery: a critical review. J Psychosom Res 1996;41(1):13–30.
8. Demeure MJ, Fain MJ. The elderly surgical patient and postoperative delirium. J Am Coll Surg 2006;203(5):752–7.
9. Kazmierski J, Kowman M, Banach M, et al. The use of DSM-IV and ICD-10 criteria and diagnostic scales for delirium among cardiac surgery patients: results from the IPDACS study. J Neuropsychiatry Clin Neurosci 2010;22(4): 426–32.
10. Inouye SK, Charpentier PA. Precipitating factors for delirium in hospitalized elderly persons. Predictive model and interrelationship with baseline vulnerability. JAMA 1996;275(11):852–7.
11. Schenning K, Deiner S. Postoperative delirium: a review of risk factors and tools of prediction. Curr Anesthesiol Rep 2014;5(1):48–56.
12. American Geriatrics Society Expert Panel on Postoperative Delirium in Older Adults. American geriatrics society abstracted clinical practice guideline for postoperative delirium in older adults. J Am Geriatr Soc 2015;63(1):142–50.
13. Chow WB, Rosenthal RA, Merkow RP, et al. Optimal preoperative assessment of the geriatric surgical patient: a best practices guideline from the American College of Surgeons National Surgical Quality Improvement Program and the American Geriatrics Society. J Am Coll Surg 2012;215(4):453–66.
14. Duppils GS, Wikblad K. Acute confusional states in patients undergoing hip surgery. A prospective observation study. Gerontology 2000;46(1):36–43.
15. American Psychiatric Association. Diagnostic and statistical manual of mental disorders. Arlington (VA): American Psychiatric Association; 2013.
16. Meagher DJ, Leonard M, Donnelly S, et al. A longitudinal study of motor subtypes in delirium: relationship with other phenomenology, etiology, medication exposure and prognosis. J Psychosom Res 2011;71(6):395–403.
17. Robinson TN, Raeburn CD, Tran ZV, et al. Postoperative delirium in the elderly: risk factors and outcomes. Ann Surg 2009;249(1):173–8.
18. Inouye SK, van Dyck CH, Alessi CA, et al. Clarifying confusion: the confusion assessment method. A new method for detection of delirium. Ann Intern Med 1990;113(12):941–8.
19. Albert MS, Levkoff SE, Reilly C, et al. The delirium symptom interview: an interview for the detection of delirium symptoms in hospitalized patients. J Geriatr Psychiatry Neurol 1992;5(1):14–21.
20. Ely EW, Margolin R, Francis J, et al. Evaluation of delirium in critically ill patients: validation of the Confusion Assessment Method for the Intensive Care Unit (CAM-ICU). Crit Care Med 2001;29(7):1370–9.

21. Gaudreau JD, Gagnon P, Harel F, et al. Fast, systematic, and continuous delirium assessment in hospitalized patients: the nursing delirium screening scale. J Pain Symptom Manage 2005;29(4):368–75.
22. Bergeron N, Dubois MJ, Dumont M, et al. Intensive care delirium screening checklist: evaluation of a new screening tool. Intensive Care Med 2001;27(5): 859–64.
23. Neelon VJ, Champagne MT, Carlson JR, et al. The NEECHAM confusion scale: construction, validation, and clinical testing. Nurs Res 1996;45(6):324–30.
24. Maldonado JR. Neuropathogenesis of delirium: review of current etiologic theories and common pathways. Am J Geriatr Psychiatry 2013;21(12):1190–222.
25. Hshieh TT, Fong TG, Marcantonio ER, et al. Cholinergic deficiency hypothesis in delirium: a synthesis of current evidence. J Gerontol A Biol Sci Med Sci 2008; 63(7):764–72.
26. Dantzer R, Konsman JP, Bluthe RM, et al. Neural and humoral pathways of communication from the immune system to the brain: parallel or convergent? Auton Neurosci 2000;85(1–3):60–5.
27. Munhoz CD, Sorrells SF, Caso JR, et al. Glucocorticoids exacerbate lipopolysaccharide-induced signaling in the frontal cortex and hippocampus in a dose-dependent manner. J Neurosci 2010;30(41):13690–8.
28. Cerejeira J, Firmino H, Vaz-Serra A, et al. The neuroinflammatory hypothesis of delirium. Acta Neuropathol 2010;119(6):737–54.
29. Capri M, Yani SL, Chattat R, et al. Pre-Operative, High-IL-6 Blood Level is a Risk Factor of Post-Operative Delirium Onset in Old Patients. Front Endocrinol (Lausanne) 2014;5:173.
30. Cape E, Hall RJ, van Munster BC, et al. Cerebrospinal fluid markers of neuroinflammation in delirium: a role for interleukin-1beta in delirium after hip fracture. J Psychosom Res 2014;77(3):219–25.
31. Cerejeira J, Lagarto L, Mukaetova-Ladinska EB. The immunology of delirium. Neuroimmunomodulation 2014;21(2–3):72–8.
32. Cerejeira J, Batista P, Nogueira V, et al. The stress response to surgery and postoperative delirium: evidence of hypothalamic-pituitary-adrenal axis hyperresponsiveness and decreased suppression of the GH/IGF-1 Axis. J Geriatr Psychiatry Neurol 2013;26(3):185–94.
33. Maldonado JR. Pathoetiological model of delirium: a comprehensive understanding of the neurobiology of delirium and an evidence-based approach to prevention and treatment. Crit Care Clin 2008;24(4):789–856, ix.
34. MacLullich AM, Ferguson KJ, Miller T, et al. Unravelling the pathophysiology of delirium: a focus on the role of aberrant stress responses. J Psychosom Res 2008;65(3):229–38.
35. Reiter RJ. Oxidative damage in the central nervous system: protection by melatonin. Prog Neurobiol 1998;56(3):359–84.
36. Robinson TN, Dunn CL, Adams JC, et al. Tryptophan supplementation and postoperative delirium–a randomized controlled trial. J Am Geriatr Soc 2014;62(9): 1764–71.
37. Palmbergen WA, van Sonderen A, Keyhan-Falsafi AM, et al. Improved perioperative neurological monitoring of coronary artery bypass graft patients reduces the incidence of postoperative delirium: the Haga Brain Care Strategy. Interact Cardiovasc Thorac Surg 2012;15(4):671–7.
38. Deiner S, Chu I, Mahanian M, et al. Prone position is associated with mild cerebral oxygen desaturation in elderly surgical patients. PLoS One 2014; 9(9):e106387.

39. Morimoto Y, Yoshimura M, Utada K, et al. Prediction of postoperative delirium after abdominal surgery in the elderly. J Anesth 2009;23(1):51–6.
40. Marcantonio ER, Flacker JM, Wright RJ, et al. Reducing delirium after hip fracture: a randomized trial. J Am Geriatr Soc 2001;49(5):516–22.
41. Inouye SK, Bogardus ST Jr, Charpentier PA, et al. A multicomponent intervention to prevent delirium in hospitalized older patients. N Engl J Med 1999;340(9): 669–76.
42. Vaurio LE, Sands LP, Wang Y, et al. Postoperative delirium: the importance of pain and pain management. Anesth Analg 2006;102(4):1267–73.
43. Sieber FE, Zakriya KJ, Gottschalk A, et al. Sedation depth during spinal anesthesia and the development of postoperative delirium in elderly patients undergoing hip fracture repair. Mayo Clin Proc 2010;85(1):18–26.
44. Chan MT, Cheng BC, Lee TM, et al. BIS-guided anesthesia decreases postoperative delirium and cognitive decline. J Neurosurg Anesthesiol 2013;25(1):33–42.
45. Radtke FM, Franck M, Lendner J, et al. Monitoring depth of anaesthesia in a randomized trial decreases the rate of postoperative delirium but not postoperative cognitive dysfunction. Br J Anaesth 2013;110(Suppl 1):i98–105.
46. Hudetz JA, Patterson KM, Iqbal Z, et al. Ketamine attenuates delirium after cardiac surgery with cardiopulmonary bypass. J Cardiothorac Vasc Anesth 2009; 23(5):651–7.
47. Hudetz JA, Pagel PS. Neuroprotection by ketamine: a review of the experimental and clinical evidence. J Cardiothorac Vasc Anesth 2010;24(1):131–42.
48. Avidan MS, Fritz BA, Maybrier HR, et al. The Prevention of Delirium and Complications Associated with Surgical Treatments (PODCAST) study: protocol for an international multicentre randomised controlled trial. BMJ Open 2014;4(9):e005651.
49. Larsen KA, Kelly SE, Stern TA, et al. Administration of olanzapine to prevent postoperative delirium in elderly joint-replacement patients: a randomized, controlled trial. Psychosomatics 2010;51(5):409–18.
50. van den Boogaard M, Schoonhoven L, van Achterberg T, et al. Haloperidol prophylaxis in critically ill patients with a high risk for delirium. Crit Care 2013;17(1):R9.
51. Wang W, Li HL, Wang DX, et al. Haloperidol prophylaxis decreases delirium incidence in elderly patients after noncardiac surgery: a randomized controlled trial*. Crit Care Med 2012;40(3):731–9.
52. Administration US FDA. FDA requests boxed warnings on older class of antipsychotic drugs. 2008. 2015 (January/30). Available at: http://www.fda.gov/News Events/Newsroom/PressAnnouncements/2008/ucm116912.htm.
53. Page VJ, Ely EW, Gates S, et al. Effect of intravenous haloperidol on the duration of delirium and coma in critically ill patients (Hope-ICU): a randomised, double-blind, placebo-controlled trial. Lancet Respir Med 2013;1(7):515–23.
54. Schrijver EJ, de Vries OJ, Verburg A, et al. Efficacy and safety of haloperidol prophylaxis for delirium prevention in older medical and surgical at-risk patients acutely admitted to hospital through the emergency department: study protocol of a multicenter, randomised, double-blind, placebo-controlled clinical trial. BMC Geriatr 2014;14:96.
55. Stoicea N, McVicker S, Quinones A, et al. Delirium-biomarkers and genetic variance. Front Pharmacol 2014;5:75.
56. Deiner S, Lin H, Bodansky D, et al. Do Stress Markers and Anesthetic Technique Predict Delirium in the Elderly. Dement Geriatr Cogn Disord 2014;38(5–6):366–74.
57. Leung JM, Sands LP, Wang Y, et al. Apolipoprotein E e4 allele increases the risk of early postoperative delirium in older patients undergoing noncardiac surgery. Anesthesiology 2007;107(3):406–11.

58. van Munster BC, Korevaar JC, Zwinderman AH, et al. The association between delirium and the apolipoprotein E epsilon 4 allele: new study results and a meta-analysis. Am J Geriatr Psychiatry 2009;17(10):856–62.
59. Bryson GL, Wyand A, Wozny D, et al. A prospective cohort study evaluating associations among delirium, postoperative cognitive dysfunction, and apolipoprotein E genotype following open aortic repair. Can J Anaesth 2011;58(3): 246–55.

Postoperative Cognitive Dysfunction

Minding the Gaps in Our Knowledge of a Common Postoperative Complication in the Elderly

Miles Berger, MD, PhD*, Jacob W. Nadler, MD, PhD,
Jeffrey Browndyke, PhD, Niccolo Terrando, PhD,
Vikram Ponnusamy, BA, Harvey Jay Cohen, MD,
Heather E. Whitson, MD, MHS, Joseph P. Mathew, MD, MHSc, MBA

KEYWORDS

- Post-operative cognitive dysfunction • Post-operative cognitive decline
- Post-operative cognitive improvement • Elderly • Anesthesia • Surgery

KEY POINTS

- Postoperative cognitive dysfunction (POCD) is a syndrome of cognitive dysfunction following anesthesia and surgery, which likely has myriad causes.
- As an increasing number of elderly patients undergo surgery and anesthesia each year, optimizing postoperative cognitive function and preventing/treating POCD are major public health issues.
- POCD is associated with impaired quality of life, increased exit from the workforce, and increased mortality after surgery.
- POCD can be conceptualized as a lack of cognitive resilience in the face of perioperative stress.

Ever since Bedford's[1] seminal *Lancet* case series in 1955, we have known that perioperative care is sometimes followed by significant cognitive dysfunction. Although the safety of perioperative care has improved dramatically since 1955, the descriptions of cognitive dysfunction in that case series are eerily similar to the complaints of current patients suffering from postoperative cognitive dysfunction (POCD). POCD remains a common postoperative complication associated with significant

The authors are not supported by, nor maintain any financial interest in, any commercial activity that may be associated with the topic of this article.
Department of Anesthesiology, Duke University Medical Center, Duke South, Orange Zone, Room 4317, Durham, NC 27710, USA
* Corresponding author.
E-mail address: miles.berger@duke.edu

Anesthesiology Clin 33 (2015) 517–550
http://dx.doi.org/10.1016/j.anclin.2015.05.008   anesthesiology.theclinics.com

morbidity and even mortality, especially among elderly patients. There has been a great deal of interest in and controversy about POCD, from how it is measured, to how long it lasts, to its precise implications for patients. This interest and controversy is reflected partly in the increasing number of articles published on this subject (shown in **Fig. 1**). Recent work has also suggested surgery may be associated with cognitive improvement in some patients,[2–4] termed postoperative cognitive improvement (POCI). As the number of surgeries performed worldwide approaches 250 million per year[5] (with an increasing number in elderly patients), optimizing postoperative cognitive function and preventing/treating POCD are major public health issues. In this article, we review the literature on POCD and POCI, and discuss current research challenges in this area.

A DESCRIPTION OF POSTOPERATIVE COGNITIVE DYSFUNCTION AND POSTOPERATIVE COGNITIVE IMPROVEMENT
What Is Postoperative Cognitive Dysfunction?

POCD is a syndrome defined by a drop in cognitive performance on a set of neuropsychological tests from before to after surgery. Unlike delirium, this means that POCD cannot be diagnosed unless a patient has undergone formal neuropsychological testing before *and* after surgery, which typically does not happen outside a research setting. Partly as a result of this, there is no *International Classification of Diseases, 10th Revision* code for POCD, and it is not listed as a diagnosis in the *Diagnostic and Statistical Manual of Mental Disorders, Fifth Edition* (DSM-V). However, the utility of the DSM-V as a nosologic tool has been questioned recently by many, including the head of the American National Institute of Mental Health.[6] Thus, the fact that POCD is not listed in the DMS-V is of questionable import.

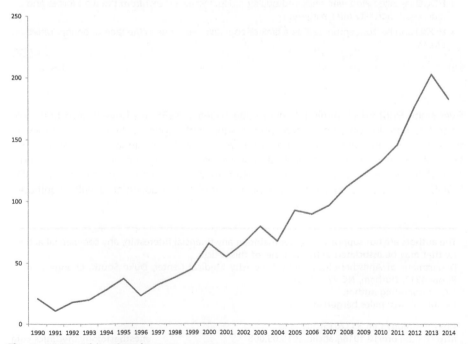

Fig. 1. POCD publications by year.

Neuropsychological testing for POCD typically includes tests that assess multiple cognitive domains (**Table 1**). Individual subtest scores are then grouped together by factor analysis or by an a priori understanding of which tests measure which cognitive domains (as described in **Table 1**). Depending on the study, anywhere from 4 to 8 cognitive domains have been used,[7,8] although simpler tests such as the Mini-Mental State Examination (MMSE) also can detect long-term postoperative cognitive changes.[9] Postoperative testing is typically performed after the acute effects of surgery and the immediate postoperative period have dissipated (ie, at least 1 week after surgery).[10] A threshold is typically set for either a drop in overall cognitive performance (the mean of the individual cognitive domain scores), or for a drop in performance in a single cognitive domain. Patients scoring below such a preset threshold are then defined as having POCD. There is no clear agreement on how low such a POCD cut-off/threshold should be set (eg, 1.0 SD, or 1.5, or 2.0 SDs).[10] There also has been disagreement over how to classify patients who drop below the preset threshold in one domain, but who show cognitive improvement in other domains.[11,12] Such patients may even show overall improvement in their composite cognitive index, even though they may meet POCD criteria (if POCD is defined as a drop below threshold in any individual cognitive domain).

Most patients typically improve their performance on these tests over repeated testing sessions due to a learning or practice effect, which makes a drop in performance all the more striking. However, this also makes it difficult to determine the true level of postoperative performance drop, because the observed postoperative performance may thus reflect both postoperative deficits and practice-related improvements. Practice effects can be mitigated by using cognitive tests with equivalent alternate forms, such that one form is used at presurgical baseline and alternate forms are used for subsequent postoperative evaluation (see **Table 1** for tests with available alternate forms). In addition to practice effects, each cognitive test has its own inherent test-retest variability, which can affect the interpretation of any postoperative cognitive change.[13] Simple change scores in performance from a patient's presurgical baseline do not take practice effects or other issues like test-retest reliability, floor/ceiling effects, or regression to the mean into account. Reliable change index (RCI) methods has been developed that can account for these effects.[14,15] The RCI is typically defined as the pretest to posttest change in a study subject minus the average pretest to posttest change among control subjects, divided by the SD of the change in pretest to posttest scores among nonsurgical controls.[16] The RCI method may have higher sensitivity and specificity for detecting POCD than other statistical methods.[16] However, unless there are published test-retest data over an equivalent time interval in age-matched individuals, the RCI method requires collecting data from nonsurgical controls at the same times as surgical patients.

The RCI method also allows one to define clinical significance thresholds for POCD, because the RCI method generates z-scores with an assumed normal distribution. An RCI score range of ±1.645, relative to a normal distribution, means that 90% of obtained change scores would fall within this range. Outliers would thus fall either in the upper or lower 5% tails of the distribution by chance. Early Alzheimer disease (AD), also known as mild cognitive impairment (MCI), is often diagnosed by a less-stringent measure of cognitive decline relative to normative performance expectations (eg, z-score drop of at least 1.5[17]). Thus, the strict −1.645 RCI criterion for clinical change significance may be excessively stringent, and may miss POCD cases that are functionally relevant to patients. There is currently no consensus among neuropsychologists of statistical method (such as an RCI) and/or threshold that should be used, and how many cognitive domains must show a decline to make the diagnosis of POCD.[10]

Table 1
Recommended neuropsychological measures for the detection and characterization of postoperative cognitive dysfunction

Core Domain	Component Cognitive Process	Measure	Description	Brain Regions/Circuits Involved in Task[b]
Global	Multiple	Montreal Cognitive Assessment (MoCA)	The MoCA is a brief cognitive screening measure tapping multiple cognitive domains, including brief assessment of memory and orientation. The screening measure is freely available (www.mocatest.org) and has the advantage of multiple alternate forms, which can help in preventing overestimation of POCD recovery secondary to simple re-administration practice effects. *Administration Time:* Variable, with ~15 min average.[124,125]	Multiple tasks, n/a.
Executive function	Simple attention	Digit Span Forward Subtest from Wechsler Adult Intelligence Scale – 3rd Revision (WAIS-III)	The Digit Span Forward subtest from the WAIS-III is a simple auditory-verbal attention task, in which a participant is asked to attend to and immediately repeat a series of serially presented digits that increase in total span as the test progresses. *Administration Time:* Variable, with ~5–10 min average.	Right dorsolateral prefrontal cortex[126]
	Complex attention (working memory)	Digit Span - Backward Subtest from Wechsler Adult Intelligence Scale – 3rd Revision (WAIS-III) or Letter-Number Sequencing Subtest from WAIS-III	The Digit Span Backward (or Letter-Number Sequencing) subtest from the WAIS-III engages both simple attention and working memory skills. Participants are instructed to attend to a series of verbally presented digits of increasing total length, but rather than respond verbatim, participants are instructed to repeat the presented digits in reverse order. In the alternate Letter-Number Sequencing subtest from the WAIS-III, participants are presented with randomized series of digits and letters of the alphabet of increasing length and asked to respond to a particular series with all digits in ascending order and all letters in alphabetical order.[126,127] *Administration Time:* Variable, with ~5–10 min average.	Right dorsolateral prefrontal cortex[126]

Response inhibition	Stroop Color Word Test	A time-limited test of the ability to inhibit a pre-potent response, known to be sensitive to medial prefrontal lobe dysfunction. The Stroop Color Word Test requires participants to read a series of color words (red, green, blue), then name the color ink of a series of X characters, after which an inhibition trial is given in which the participant is asked to name the color ink of a series of color words that are in opposition to the ink color (eg, the word blue printed in red ink). The natural tendency of participants is to say the word as printed rather than the ink color; hence the sensitivity of the measure to response inhibition skills. *Administration Time:* 3–4 min.	Anterior cingulate cortex (ACC), right inferior frontal gyrus, and cerebellum[128]
Mental flexibility	Trail Making A & B Test[a]	The timed Trail Making A subtest requires participants to connect a series of numbered circles distributed on a piece of paper in ascending numerical order, whereas the Trail Making B subtest has both letters of the alphabet and numbers in circles that then must be connected in alternating ascending order (eg, 1-A-2-B-3-C…). Trail Making A & B tests should be administered in immediate succession, as the Trail Making A subtest is necessary for familiarization of general subtest B task requirements. Independent administration of Trail Making B test only may result in overestimation of POCD severity.[129,130] *Administration Time:* Variable with 5-min timed maximum for each subtest.	Medial temporal lobe[130], left-sided dorsolateral and medial frontal cortex[165]
Verbal fluency	Controlled Oral Word Association Test (COWA) from the Multilingual Aphasia Examination (MAE)[a]	A lexical verbal fluency task known to be dependent on pre-Broca area function in the language dominant brain hemisphere. This test also requires retention of task rules for proper performance. Participants say as many words as they can retrieve that start with a particular consonant with 1-min given for 3 different consonants (eg, C, F, L). Participants are asked to not use proper nouns or the same word with different endings (eg, eat, eating). *Administration Time:* 3 min.	Posterior part of the left inferior prefrontal cortex (LIPC); category fluency task activates anterior LIPC and right inferior prefrontal cortex[131,132]

(continued on next page)

Table 1
(continued)

Core Domain	Component Cognitive Process	Measure	Description	Brain Regions/Circuits Involved in Task[b]
Learning and memory	Auditory-verbal learning & memory	Hopkins Verbal Learning Test, Revised (HVLT-R)[a]	An auditory-verbal, list-learning, and memory task that involves the presentation of 12 various categorically related item words (eg, gemstones, furniture) that are then immediately recalled by the participant. Participants are given the opportunity to learn the list of words over a series of 3 repeated presentations, then after a 25-min delay, participants are assessed for delayed recall and recognition memory for the primary word list items. Scored items include total recall, delayed recall, percent retention (after delay), and recognition discrimination index. *Administration Time*: 35 min timed (includes 25-min delay).	Left ventrolateral prefrontal cortex[133]
	Visual learning & memory	Brief Visuospatial Learning Test, Revised[a]	A visuospatial learning and memory test analog to the HVLT-R. Six simple line drawings are presented in a 2 × 3 array on a single piece of paper and participants are allowed a brief period to study the figures, after which they are asked to reproduce as many figures in their proper locations as they can on a blank sheet of paper. Three learning trials of the 6 line drawings are conducted. There is a 25-min delay, after which participants are asked to recall as many figures in their locations as possible. Delayed recognition for the same line drawings is also conducted. Scored items are the same as the HVLT-R (eg, total recall, delayed recall).[134] *Administration Time*: 45 min timed (includes 25-min delay)	

		Test	Description	Brain regions
Visuospatial functioning	Visuomotor integration	Digit Symbol Coding Test from the Wechsler Adult Intelligence Scale–3rd Revision (WAIS-III)	The Digit Symbol Coding Test requires participants to use a symbol/number key at the top of a printed page as a guide to determine the appropriate missing symbols for a large array of unmatched numbers below the test key. The task is timed and the scored response is the total number of correct symbol/number pairs completed by the participant within 120 s. *Administration Time:* 5 min.	Corpus callosum, internal capsule[135]; anterior cingulate gyrus, left prefrontal gyrus, and inferior parietal lobe[136]
	Complex visuospatial perception	Hooper Visual Organizational Test (HVOT)	HVOT performance is known to be dependent on bilateral parietal and temporal-occipital cortex functioning and involves participants' mental integration and naming of common objects presented in a spatially scattered puzzle piece–like format. Proper execution of the task requires participants to mentally rotate and connect partial stimuli pieces into a whole to form a perceptual gestalt. *Administration Time:* Variable, with ~10–12 min average.	Superior parietal lobules, ventral temporal-occipital cortex, and posterior visual association areas, frontal eye fields, left dorsolateral prefrontal cortex[137]
Psychomotor function	Manual dexterity & motor speed	Lafayette Grooved Pegboard Test	A manipulative dexterity and motor speed test that involves the insertion of small milled keylike pins into randomly rotated matching holes arranged in a 5 × 5 array. Each hand is evaluated separately with a score reflecting the total time to complete insertion of all 25 pegs for each hand. *Administration Time:* Variable, with ~5 min average.	Nigrostriatal dopamine function[138]

[a] Recommended measures with readily available alternate, equivalent forms.

[b] Brain regions associated with test performance by functional MRI, other brain regions may also be involved. For further discussion of the uses and limitations of fMRI technology, see Refs. [139,140]

Although POCD has been defined by the statistical results of cognitive tests, multiple investigators have found that it is also associated with impairments in quality of life,[18] increased exit from the workforce,[19] and increased mortality after surgery.[19,20] Thus, POCD can be conceptualized as a lack of resilience in the face of perioperative stress,[21] which is associated with impairments in multiple aspects of life. This conceptual model raises the question of whether POCD also may be associated with impairments in social relationships, increased physical frailty, decreased sexual interest and/or performance, and deficits in other aspects of life; these are important questions to be addressed by future studies (see **Table 4**).

How Long Does Postoperative Cognitive Dysfunction Last?

Aside from this disagreement over how POCD diagnosis is defined, it is also unclear how long it may last. This issue is difficult to address for several reasons. First, it is ethically unreasonable and practically impossible to randomize patients to surgery and anesthesia (vs placebo treatment). Without a nonsurgical control group, though, it is unclear how much of the cognitive dysfunction in surgical patients is truly due to anesthesia, surgery, and perioperative care.[22] The initial rapid drop in cognition seen in patients with POCD occurs much more rapidly than normal age-related cognitive decline.[20,23]

Matched cohort study designs can attempt to provide nonsurgical control groups for comparison, but such study designs are nonrandomized and thus potentially confounded by the fact that surgical patients may be intrinsically different from nonsurgical controls. Nonetheless, several studies have compared the incidence of cognitive dysfunction in surgical patients and nonsurgical controls.[23,24] In the International Study of Post-Operative Cognitive Dysfunction (ISPOCD), statistically significant differences in the incidence of cognitive dysfunction were found between surgical patients and nonsurgical controls at 1 week and 3 months after surgery,[23] but no difference was seen at 1 year after surgery. In a prospective matched cohort study, however, greater cognitive dysfunction was seen in surgical patients than nonsurgical controls even at 1 year after surgery.[24] A retrospective study by Avidan and colleagues[25] found no difference in the cognitive decline trajectory between noncardiac surgical patients and matched controls over a period of up to several years (median of 3.1 years of follow-up in surgical patients). However, the 2 largest studies to examine this issue both found that patients who have gone through anesthesia and surgery are at an increased risk of developing dementia years later.[26,27] Taken together, these data suggest that POCD after noncardiac surgery typically lasts months or even up to a year, but does not exclude the possibility that it may last longer in some cases. Whether perioperative care and/or POCD are linked to a long-term risk of developing dementia remains an important question for future prospective studies (see **Table 4**).[28]

After cardiac surgery, Newman and colleagues[7] found an overall cognitive trajectory of decline up to 5 years later. Interestingly, cognitive dysfunction in the early postoperative period was a predictor of cognitive decline 5 years later,[7] raising the possibility that long-term cognitive decline after cardiac surgery may be caused by insults sustained during the perioperative period. This view is challenged, however, by data from Selnes and colleagues,[8,29,30] who found no difference in the long-term cognitive trajectory (at 3 or 6 years after surgery) in patients with coronary artery disease (CAD) who underwent cardiac surgery versus control patients with CAD who did not undergo cardiac surgery. Similarly, patients with CAD who underwent off-pump coronary artery bypass grafting (CABG) had similar cognitive outcomes as patients with CAD who underwent percutaneous coronary intervention.[31] Thus, there is clearly long-term cognitive decline that occurs over years in older patients with CAD, but this long-term decline appears to be largely due to patient factors (such as preexisting neurovascular disease) rather than procedural factors (such as cardiac surgery, cardiopulmonary bypass, or anesthesia itself[32]). This interpretation need not imply that the mechanisms of cognitive decline are identical in patients with CAD treated surgically versus medically, though.[33] Taken together, these data suggest that, as in the case of POCD after noncardiac surgery, POCD after cardiac surgery may last from weeks to several months. However, the current data do not rule out the possibility that POCD after cardiac surgery may last longer in some cases.

In asking how long POCD may last, it is important to note that POCD is a syndrome rather than a disease caused by a single underlying pathophysiologic process. In this sense, POCD is more akin to a fever than influenza. Although a recent study suggested that POCD is independent of surgical procedure or anesthetic drug choice on a population level,[34] there are likely some patients who experience POCD due to specific intraoperative or perioperative factors, and the duration of POCD likely depends on its specific etiology. For example, the fifth patient in Bedford's case report[1] was described as "an intelligent and active man—mentally normal in every way" before surgery, but after he was "unable to recognize his relations and remained unaware of his surroundings" even up to 18 months after surgery. This severe POCD was likely related to the fact that this patient's "blood pressure fell to unrecordable levels for about 15 minutes" during surgery.[1] There is considerable evidence that prolonged cerebral hypoperfusion can cause cerebral ischemic damage and result in lifelong neurocognitive deficits. Thus, it is likely that this patient's postoperative cognitive dysfunction was caused by intraoperative hypotension, and that it lasted the rest of this patient's life (this could be conceptualized as the bottom trajectory in **Fig. 2**). Although this is a somewhat extreme case (intraoperative periods of undetectable blood pressure lasting more than 15 minutes are currently extremely rare, except in

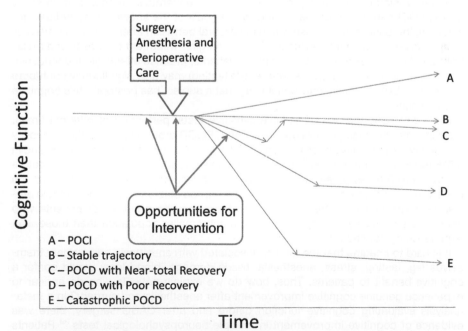

Fig. 2. Potential cognitive trajectories following surgery.

deep hypothermic circulatory arrest cases), this example makes the point that the duration of POCD depends on its etiology. This should come as no surprise. The length, severity, and outcome of any syndrome depends on its cause; a fever caused by a cold virus is likely to have a shorter duration and better outcome than one caused by gram-negative rod sepsis.

We believe that the question of how long POCD lasts, as opposed to how long other types of cognitive deficits may last, is largely irrelevant for individual patients though. If a patient is suffering from cognitive decline, in most cases he or she (and family members) are unlikely to care what percentage of the cognitive decline may be attributable to perioperative care, versus what percentage may have occurred in the absence of perioperative care. Furthermore, there is no way to calculate these percentages on an individual patient basis, and even if we could calculate these percentages on an individual patient basis, it would be therapeutically irrelevant: there is currently no specific treatment for POCD that differs from that for any other age-related cognitive disorder. Nonetheless, patients may ask preoperatively what their risk of POCD is, and how long it may last. At a population level, we believe that current data suffice to tell patients that most cases of POCD resolve within months after both noncardiac and cardiac surgery, although it is impossible to tell how long any individual case of POCD will last. It is important to emphasize during preoperative counseling that POCD has more than one potential underlying cause, and if it develops, the course and prognosis will depend on its cause(s).

What Is Postoperative Cognitive Improvement?

Although much of the focus has been on patients who experience a worsening of cognitive performance after anesthesia and surgery, the same neuropsychological testing demonstrates that some patients improve their cognitive performance after their procedure. This enhancement may reflect a genuine improvement in cognitive function, or simply the slowing or reversal of a preoperative deterioration. In some cases, POCI can be directly attributed to the goals of the specific surgery itself, for example, the postoperative restoration of cerebral perfusion after carotid endarterectomy,[35] the removal of a brain lesion,[36] or the surgical treatment of obesity and metabolic syndrome.[3,4] However, even in these patients, practice effects (ie, the tendency for test performance to improve with repeat testing) may also significantly contribute to the probability of mistakenly concluding that a subject has postoperative cognitive improvement.[37]

More generally, the use of multiple sensitive tests, performed at different times, results in great measurement variability. The ISPOCD group examined this variability and uncovered cognitive improvement in 4.2% to 8.7% of patients after 1 week and in 5.0% to 7.8% after 3 months.[38] However, in the same population, these investigators found a 3 to 6 times greater incidence of POCD, leading them to conclude that the observed "improvement" merely reflected the unpredictable variability inherent in precise neuropsychological testing. Although there may be a subset of patients who improve after surgery, it appears to be a much smaller population than those who experience dysfunction.[38]

It is hard to imagine that the factors associated with anesthesia and surgery themselves (eg, fasting, stress, anesthesia, tissue damage, blood loss) would confer a cognitive benefit to patients. Thus, how do we explain patients who do appear to experience genuine cognitive improvement after anesthesia and surgery? In a meta-analysis evaluating cognitive function before and after CABG surgery, there was evidence of cognitive improvement in multiple neuropsychological tests.[39] Patients receiving CABG also demonstrate improved physical, social, and emotional function

6 months and 1 year after surgery, including less anxiety and depression.[40] It is likely that the improvement in the cognitive function of patients who received CABG stems from this generalized improvement in overall health and quality of life, especially given the known negative effects of depression on cognitive performance.[41,42] Moreover, a successful surgery sometimes enables patients to taper or discontinue cognition-clouding medications (eg, medications for pain, sleep, or anxiety) that were used preoperatively, and may thus allow patients to improve their overall functioning. In line with this idea, even among patients who had POCD at 6 weeks after surgery, increased ability to perform instrumental activities of daily living at 6 weeks after surgery was associated improved cognition at 1 year.[2]

How Long Does Postoperative Cognitive Improvement Last?

It is unclear how long cognitive improvement would last if it results from a generalized improvement in health postoperatively. The increases in performance described previously began to appear at 3 months, and continued throughout the first year after cardiac surgery.[39] In bariatric surgery, improvements were seen 2 and 3 years later.[3,4] We hypothesize that postoperative cognitive improvement will last as long as a patient's general health and quality of life remain improved after surgery, and this is an important question for future study (see **Table 4**).

A Comparison Between Postoperative Cognitive Dysfunction and Other Medically Related/Induced Cognitive Disorders

The phenomenon of POCD has a parallel in the cognitive changes associated with cancer and chemotherapy (reviewed in Ref.[43]). Although some of the classical psychological sequelae of cancer diagnosis (including depression, anxiety, fatigue) are independently associated with alterations in cognitive function, it remains difficult to untangle the pathophysiology of cancer-related cognitive impairment (CRCI) because several chemotherapeutic agents have direct neurotoxic actions (reviewed in Ref.[44]) and modulate interactions between the immune system and brain.[45] Although CRCI appears to occur more frequently than POCD, the 2 syndromes share many of the same characteristics, including demographics, biological factors, and time courses. As in the case of POCD, older patients and those with lower levels of pretreatment cognitive reserve experience the greatest reductions in performance from CRCI.[46,47] These impairments occur in multiple cognitive domains, reach a nadir shortly after cancer treatment, and then gradually return toward baseline.[48] Additionally, many of the proposed mechanisms of "chemo-brain" are the same ones proposed in the POCD literature (discussed later in this article). Patients subjectively report greater deficits than are seen in objective neuropsychological testing in both POCD and CRCI,[49,50] which suggests that the neurocognitive tests used in CRCI and POCD testing do not pick up the full intensity of the cognitive impairments that patients themselves experience. Unfortunately, many of the same methodological problems (eg, inability to randomize, variation between studies in criteria used to define cognitive impairment, practice-related effects) affect studies on both POCD and CRCI.

WHO IS AT RISK FOR DEVELOPING POSTOPERATIVE COGNITIVE DYSFUNCTION?
Modifiable Risk Factors

Several studies have examined risk factors for POCD (**Tables 2** and **3** for a list of modifiable and nonmodifiable POCD risk factors, respectively). Interestingly, several studies have found that either lighter anesthetic depth or careful anesthetic depth monitoring can lower POCD rates,[51,52] which suggests that POCD may be due to

Table 2
Potentially modifiable risk factors for POCD

Risk Factor	Effect Size	Study Design	Reference
Bispectral index (EEG) guided anesthetic care (vs routine care)	OR 0.92 (0.66–1.29) at 1 wk $P = .06$ OR 0.62 (0.39–0.97) at 3 mo $P = .02$	RCT	51
	18.1% vs 23.9% at 7 d $P = .062$ 8% vs 10.3% at 3 mo $P = .372$	RCT	52
Fentanyl dosage	Low (10 µg/kg) vs high-dose fentanyl (50 µg/kg), POCD rates 23.6% vs 13.7% at 1 wk, respectively, $P = .03$. NS at 3 and 12 mo.	RCT	141
Ketamine treatment	2 SD drop in overall cognition in 7/26 ketamine group vs 21/26 patients, $P<.001$	RCT	107
Lidocaine vs no lidocaine	POCD 18.6% vs 40%, $P = .028$	RCT	142
	Neurocognitive deficit 45.8% vs 40.7% at 10 wk $P = .577$ 35.2% vs 37.7% at 25 wk $P = .710$	RCT	143
	45.5% vs 45.7%, $P = .97$	RCT	66
Magnesium sulfate infusion	Multivariate OR for low dose 0.09 (0.02–0.50), $P = .01$; OR for high dose 0.45 (0.16–1.33), $P = .15$	RCT	144
	44.4% vs 44.9%, $P = .93$	RCT	106
Piracetam vs no piracetam	Overall cognitive function preoperative 0.06 ± 1.02 vs -0.06 ± 0.99 postoperative -0.65 ± 0.93 vs -1.38 ± 1.11, $P<.0005$	RCT	145
Intraoperative steroid treatment	No vs low-dose vs high-dose dexamethasone POCD 22.3% vs 20.6% vs 31.4%, $P = .003$	RCT	110
	RR 1.87 (0.90–3.88) at 1 mo $P = .09$ RR 1.98 (0.61–6.40) at 1 y $P = .24$	RCT	109
Postoperative delirium[a]	Multivariate OR 9.58 (4.62–19.9), $P<.001$	RCT	51
	POCD vs no POCD[b] 1.5% vs 1.1% at discharge $P = .046$ 6.7% vs 5.6% at 3 mo $P = .373$	Prospective cohort study	20
	Delirium vs no delirium MMSE scores: 24.1 vs 27.4 at 1 mo $P<.001$ 25.2 vs 27.2 at 1 y $P<.001$	Prospective cohort study	9

Postoperative infection[a]	Univariate OR 2.17 (1.50–3.15), $P = .001$	RCT	51
Postoperative respiratory complication[a]	Univariate OR 1.69 (1.01–2.89), $P = .02$	RCT	51
Metabolic syndrome[a]	POCD vs no POCD 43.3% vs 26.7%, $P<.02$	Prospective cohort study	127
Cigarette abuse	Multivariate OR 2.04 (1.11–3.74), $P = .022$ NS	RCT Prospective cohort study	146 23
Diabetes[a]	Multivariate OR 2.34 (1.22–4.51), $P = .01$ POCD vs no POCD 40% vs 19.2%, $P = .021$	Prospective cohort study Prospective cohort study	11 104
	Multivariate linear regression, parameter estimate 0.031 (−0.111–0.172), $P = .671$	RCT	66
Duration of anesthesia	OR 1.1 (1.0–1.3), $P = .01$ POCD vs no POCD at 3 mo	Prospective cohort study Prospective cohort study	23 20
	215.0 ± 92.8 vs 211.5 ± 103.2 min duration, $P = .52$ POCD vs no POCD 5.6 ± 1.5 vs 5.0 ± 1.2, $P = .026$	Prospective cohort study	104
	POCD vs no POCD 4.6 ± 1.5 vs 3.8 ± 0.8, $P = .001$	Prospective cohort study	147
Benzodiazepines before surgery	OR 0.4 (0.2–1.0), $P = .03$	Prospective cohort study	23
Duration of hospital stay	POCD vs no POCD 6.6 ± 16.3 vs 4.8 ± 5.9 at discharge $P = .0003$ Multivariate OR 1.03 (1.00–1.05) at 3 mo $P = .2479$	Prospective cohort study	20
Duration of surgery	POCD vs no POCD 4.7 ± 0.9 vs 4.2 ± 1.0, $P = .01$	Prospective cohort study	104
Anesthetic type (general vs regional)	Mean Difference −0.08 (−0.17–0.01), $P = .094$ General vs nongeneral anesthesia, OR 1.34 (0.95–1.93), $P = .26$	Meta-analysis Meta-analysis	56 55

(continued on next page)

Table 2
(continued)

Risk Factor	Effect Size	Study Design	Reference
Bispectral index and cerebral oxygenation monitoring	1 wk mild Fisher's exact test $P = .018$ 1 wk moderate, Pearson $P = .037$ 1 wk severe, Fisher exact test $P = .12$ 12 wk mild χ^2 test $P = .02$ 12 wk moderate χ^2 test $P = .85$ 12 wk severe χ^2 test $P = .65$ 1 y mild χ^2 test $P = .015$ 1 y moderate χ^2 test $P = .02$ 1 y severe Fisher exact test $P = .36$	RCT	[24]
Postoperative copeptin levels[a]	OR 28.814 (7.131–116.425), $P<.001$	Prospective cohort study	[104]
Peripheral inflammatory markers[a]	S-100β standardized mean difference 1.377 (0.423–2.331), $P = .005$ IL-6 standardized mean difference 1.614 (0.603–2.624), $P = .002$	Meta-analysis	[148]
Off-pump vs on-pump cardiac surgery	Standardized cognitive change score 0.19 vs 0.13 at 3 mo $P = .03$ 0.19 vs 0.12 at 1 y $P = .09$	RCT	[149]
	Off-pump vs on-pump vs nonsurgical cardiac comparison vs healthy heart comparison MMSE 27.7 ± 2.0 vs 27.6 ± 2.4 vs 27.9 ± 2.0 vs 28.5 ± 1.9 at baseline $P<.01$ 28.5 ± 1.8 vs 27.4 ± 2.5 vs 28.0 ± 2.3 vs 28.6 ± 1.7 at 6 y $P<.01$ 62% vs 53% at postoperative day 4, $P = .50$; 39% vs 14% at 3 mo $P = .04$	Prospective longitudinal study	[8]
		RCT	[150]
Perfusion pressure (in cardiac surgery)	MMSE score drop 48 h after surgery, in low pressure vs high pressure: 3.9 ± 6.5 vs 1.1 ± 1.9, $P = .012$	RCT	[151]
r_{SO_2} Desaturation score >3000	Multivariate OR 2.22 (1.11–4.45), $P = .024$	RCT	[146]
Hemodilution (in CPB cases)	Age × hemodilution interaction, $P = .03$	RCT, stopped early	[152]

Hyperglycemia (ie, glucose >200 mg/dL at any point during CPB cases)	Associated with POCD in nondiabetic patients, N = 380, OR = 1.85 (95% CI 1.12–3.04), $P = .017$; NS ($P = .81$) in diabetic patients, n = 145	Retrospective analysis of pooled data from multiple previous prospective studies	153
Slow rewarming vs normal rewarming (in CPB cases)	Multivariate linear regression variable estimate 0.35, $P = .047$ (favoring slow rewarming)	RCT	154
Continuous cell saver use (in CPB cases)	6% vs 15% in controls, $P = .038$ 16.7% vs 15.9% in controls, relative risk: 1.05, 95% CI 0.58–1.90 at 3 mo.	RCT RCT	155 156
Embolic load (in CPB cases)	No correlation between embolic load measured by transcranial Doppler ultrasound and POCD at 1 wk ($P = .617$) or at 3 mo ($P = .110$), n = 356 patients.	Pooled analysis of data from 2 other RCTs	102
Alpha stat vs pH stat blood gas management (in CPB cases)	27% vs 44%, $P = .047$	RCT	157
Hypothermia vs normothermia (in CPB cases)	Multivariate odds ratio 1.15 (95% CI 1.01–1.31), $P = .042$, for POCD at hospital discharge after intraoperative normothermia vs mild hypothermia.	Retrospective analysis of pooled data from 2 previous trials	158
	NS difference for POCD at 6 wk after surgery.	RCT	159
	Hypothermia vs normothermia, relative risk for POCD at 1 wk after surgery = 0.77, $P = .048$.	RCT	160
	Hypothermia vs normothermia, relative risk for POCD at 5 y after surgery = 0.66, $P = .16$.	RCT	161

Abbreviations: CI, confidence interval; CPB, cardiopulmonary bypass; EEG, electroencephalogram; MMSE, Mini-Mental State Examination; NS, not significant; OR, odds ratio; POCD, postoperative cognitive dysfunction; RCT, randomized controlled trial; RR, relative risk.

[a] Partially modifiable risk factor.
[b] Delirium during hospital stay.

Table 3
Nonmodifiable risk factors for POCD

Risk Factor	POCD vs No POCD	Study Design	Reference
Age	Multivariate OR 1.04 (1.01–1.08), P = .01	RCT	51
	Multivariate OR 1.03 (0.99–1.06), P = .1	Prospective observational study	11
	Age of patients with POCD 51.9 ± 17.3 vs no POCD 49.4 ± 16.5, measured at discharge P = .027	Prospective cohort study	20
	OR 1.03 (1.01–1.06), P = .013	Prospective cohort study	67
	OR 1.151 (1.030–1.285), P = .003	Prospective cohort study	104
	Multivariate OR 1.34 (1.01–1.78), P = .043	Prospective cohort study	147
	Multivariate OR 0.95 (0.71–1.26), P = .70	RCT	146
	Multivariate linear regression parameter estimate (for continuous cognitive change score) −0.009 (−0.012 to −0.005), P<.001	RCT	66
Educational level	Multivariate OR 0.98 (0.91–1.07), P = .67	Prospective cohort study	11
	Multivariate OR 0.84 (0.76–0.93) at 3 mo P = .0031	Prospective cohort study	20
	OR 0.9 (0.83–0.98), P = .021	Prospective cohort study	67
	Multivariable linear regression model, parameter estimate: 0.012 (−0.002–0.027), P = .098	RCT	66
Type of surgery	Minimally invasive 4% vs 34%, intra-abdominal/thoracic 21% vs 14%, orthopedic 11% vs 16% at discharge P = .001	Prospective cohort study	20
	Congenital disease 10 vs 42 / Valvular disease 32% vs 54% / Aorta disease 14% vs 20% / Tumor 2% vs 2%; P = .051 overall	Prospective cohort study	147
	NS	Prospective cohort study	23

Genetic risk alleles	CRP 1059G/C SNP OR 0.37 (0.16–0.78), $P = .013$ SELP 1087G/A SNP OR 0.51 (0.30–0.85), $P = .011$	Prospective cohort study	67
Left hippocampal volume	POCD vs no POCD 2.26 ± 0.21 vs 2.45 ± 0.15, $P<.01$	Prospective cohort study	162
Right hippocampal volume	POCD vs no POCD 2.49 ± 0.11 vs 2.62 ± 0.20, $P<.05$	Prospective cohort study	162
MCA velocity	Left MCA POCD vs no POCD 42.5 ± 5.5 vs 54.3 ± 4.4, $P<.1$ Left vs Right MCA POCD 42.5 ± 5.5 vs 56.3 ± 4.5, $P<.05$[a]	Prospective cohort study	163
Preoperative renal insufficiency	Multivariate OR 0.18 (0.04–0.75), $P = .019$	RCT	146
Previous stroke	Multivariate OR 0.30 (0.11–0.84), $P = .02$	RCT	144

Abbreviations: CRP, C-reactive protein; MCA, middle cerebral artery; NS, not significant; OR, odds ratio; POCD, postoperative cognitive dysfunction; RCT, randomized controlled trial; SELP, P-selectin; SNP, single nucleotide polymorphism.
[a] Values estimated from the bar graph in **Fig. 1**.

excessive anesthetic drug exposure in some cases. In line with these findings, a previous study found an increased rate of POCD 1 week after general versus regional anesthesia (P = .06 overall, P = .04 in an as treated analysis[53]), although there was no difference in POCD rates 3 months after surgery (P = .93). However, Silbert and colleagues[54] recently found no difference in POCD rates between patients who underwent extracorporeal shock wave lithotripsy under either general or spinal anesthesia; if anything, there was a surprising trend toward increased POCD risk in the spinal anesthesia group (P = .06, and the trial was stopped early). This suggests that general anesthesia does not increase POCD risk. These findings are particularly difficult to reconcile with those discussed previously because more than 90% of the patients in the spinal anesthesia group did not receive any intravenous sedation,[54] in contrast to many other studies in which patients randomized to receive regional anesthesia also received large doses of intravenous sedation.[53] However, the study by Silbert and colleagues[54] was nearly fourfold smaller than the study by Rasmussen and colleagues.[53] Further, the patients in the spinal anesthesia group were also 3 years older on average than those in the general anesthesia group in the study by Silbert and colleagues.[54] A meta-analysis performed on this subject in 2010 found a nonstatistically significant trend toward an increased risk of POCD after general versus regional anesthesia (odds ratio 1.34, 95% confidence interval 0.93%–1.95%, P = .26).[55] Another meta-analysis performed in 2011 also found a slight, but nonsignificant trend toward a decreased risk of POCD after regional versus general anesthesia (standardized difference in means −0.08, −0.17–0.01, P = .094,[56]). Future studies will be necessary to better understand whether there is a relationship between general anesthesia and POCD risk, and whether certain subgroups of patients (such as older patients, those with more cerebrovascular disease, or those with less cognitive reserve for other reasons) are at higher risk of developing POCD after general versus regional anesthesia (**Table 4**).

Numerous studies also have examined whether specific anesthetic drugs are tied to POCD risk. Although basic science studies have suggested differential neurotoxicity between inhaled/volatile anesthetics versus intravenous agents (reviewed in Ref.[28]), there is a paucity of well-controlled clinical studies examining this issue. For example, higher rates of cognitive decline (as measured by the MMSE) were found on 1, 2, and 3 days after surgery among 2000 patients randomized to receive inhaled versus intravenous anesthesia.[57] However, there was no MMSE test score difference between groups by 10 days after surgery in this study, there was no attempt made to ensure equivalent anesthetic depth in both groups, and patients in the inhaled group likely received a significant anesthetic overdose.[58] There was no difference in POCD rates between patients randomized to sevoflurane versus desflurane in another study, although patients who received desflurane awakened faster and had higher satisfaction scores.[59] Patients who received spinal anesthesia and isoflurane had a higher incidence of POCD than patients who received spinal anesthesia alone or spinal anesthesia plus desflurane in a pilot study.[60] It is somewhat unusual to use spinal and inhaled anesthesia together in the United States, though, which makes it hard to apply these findings to typical clinical practice. These findings are also challenged by the results of Kanbak and colleagues,[61] who found that isoflurane use was associated with improved neurocognitive function after cardiac surgery (as compared with desflurane or sevoflurane) in a similar size pilot randomized controlled trial. Schoen and colleagues[62] found that sevoflurane administration (as compared with propofol-based intravenous anesthesia) was associated with improved cognition within 1 week after on-pump cardiac surgery. In summary, the available evidence is insufficient to determine whether any specific anesthetic agent is associated with a reduced risk of POCD.

Table 4
Important questions for future research, suggestions, and challenges

Research Question	Suggested Study Design and Methods[a]	Issues/Challenges
What aspects of aging are most closely tied to POCD risk?	Cohort design, with cognitive testing and geriatric evaluations	Important to have involvement of geriatricians.
Are certain patients (ie, the elderly, or those with less cognitive reserve) at higher risk for POCD after general vs regional anesthesia?	RCT of general vs regional anesthesia with cognitive testing, stratified by age group and/or other variables	Patient recruitment, importance of minimizing sedation in the regional arm to allow for a true comparison of general vs regional anesthesia.
Is POCD associated with an increased long-term risk of dementia?	Prospective cohort with long-term follow-up, cognitive and MCI/AD/dementia screening	Need to enroll patients who may already have MCI or other baseline cognitive deficits. Large sample sizes needed to obtain sufficient power for clinically relevant effects; see Refs.[28,164] for discussion of this issue.
What is the relationship between central neuroinflammation, cerebrovascular white matter disease, AD pathology (and/or perioperative changes in these pathologic processes) and POCD?	Cohort design, cognitive testing, neuroimaging, and CSF AD and inflammatory biomarker studies	Patient recruitment.
Is POCD associated with altered functional brain connectivity?	Cohort design, cognitive testing and functional MRI scans	Patient recruitment, MRI safety issues may exclude some elderly patients with pacemakers/AICDs, metal joint replacements, and so forth.
Are there CSF biomarkers of POCD?	Cohort design, cognitive testing and CSF sampling	Patient recruitment.
Would SSRI treatment prevent POCD; improve cognitive trajectory, affect, and mood; and/or improve quality of life in patients with POCD?	RCT, cognitive testing, quality-of-life measurement, depression/anxiety and affect rating scales	Possible side effects from treatment.

(continued on next page)

Table 4
(continued)

Research Question	Suggested Study Design and Methods[a]	Issues/Challenges
Would preconditioning with ischemia or anesthetic agents help prevent POCD?	RCT	Patient recruitment.
Would physical and/or cognitive prehabilitation reduce the incidence or severity of POCD, and/or improve quality of life after surgery in the elderly?	RCT	Blinding difficult if not impossible; need to ensure patient participation in prehabilitation interventions.
How long does POCI last? Does it depend on surgery type? To what extent does POCI reflect surgically induced improvements in underlying disease processes, quality of life, and/or mental health?	Cohort design	Careful statistical analysis required to separate true POCI from test practice effects.

Abbreviations: AICD, automatic implantable cardioverter defibrillator; AD, Alzheimer disease; CSF, cerebrospinal fluid; MCI, mild cognitive impairment; POCD, postoperative cognitive dysfunction; POCI, postoperative cognitive improvement; RCT, randomized controlled trial; SSRI, selective serotonin reuptake inhibitor.
[a] For prospective study designs, it is important that all testing be completed both before and after surgery.

Several recent articles also have examined whether specific anesthetic drugs may be associated with less cognitive decline after surgery in patients with MCI (an early stage of AD). One recent study found increased rates of MCI progression 2 years later in patients who received spine surgery who were randomized to receive sevoflurane versus propofol or epidural anesthesia (n = 60 per group,[63]). Another study among patients with MCI found no difference in POCD rates among patients with MCI randomized to receive sevoflurane (n = 99) versus propofol anesthesia (n = 101) for radical rectal resection, although there was an increased rate of severe POCD in the sevoflurane-treated patients.[64] Taken together, these studies raise the possibility that propofol anesthesia (as compared with sevoflurane anesthesia) might be associated with improved postoperative cognition in patients with MCI, but further studies are necessary to examine this issue.

Nonmodifiable Risk Factors

One nonmodifiable risk factor for POCD consistently found in multiple studies is increased age[7,20,23,51,54]; POCD was present in one study more than twice as often in patients age 60 and older as in those younger than 60.[20] This association makes intuitive sense in the setting of the failed resilience model discussed previously. Older patients often have more neurovascular disease risk factors, more cerebral white matter damage, and less cognitive reserve,[65] which may place them at a higher risk of cognitive dysfunction after the stress of surgery, anesthesia, and perioperative care. Aside from age, 2 other nonmodifiable risk factors for POCD that have been found across multiple studies are fewer years of previous education and lower preoperative cognitive test scores,[20,66,67] which also fits with the idea that patients with less cognitive reserve are at higher risk of developing POCD (see **Table 3**).

Although age itself is nonmodifiable, age is also frequently associated with frailty, which is at least partly modifiable.[68–71] Numerous studies in recent years have focused on physical "prehabilitation" to decrease postoperative complications and/or improve postoperative physical function,[72–75] but to the best of our knowledge no study has evaluated whether physical and/or cognitive prehabilitation might decrease the risk of POCD. The plasticity of the human brain in response to both physical[76] and cognitive[77] exercise suggests that such interventions may help prevent and/or treat POCD. The degree to which an aging brain possesses the plasticity to benefit from such interventions is unclear, though,[78] making this is an important area for future research (see **Table 4**).

WHAT CAUSES POSTOPERATIVE COGNITIVE DYSFUNCTION?
Animal Models

Animal studies have suggested the POCD may be caused be either excessive neuroinflammation after surgery,[79] a failure to resolve inflammation,[80,81] blood-brain barrier/endothelial dysfunction,[82–84] and/or preexisting AD pathology (reviewed in Ref.[28]). Activation of the innate immune system is increasingly appreciated as an underlying factor in several neurodegenerative conditions, including AD. Using different preclinical models of non–central nervous system surgery, neuroinflammation has been repeatedly associated with behavioral dysfunction and memory deficits. Upregulation of systemic proinflammatory cytokines, including tumor necrosis factor-alpha, interleukin (IL)-1, IL-6, chemokines, and damage-associated molecular patterns, like high-mobility group box 1, have been shown to activate bone-marrow derived macrophages and contribute to the overall brain pathology after aseptic trauma.[80,81,85,86] Several mechanisms, including humoral, cellular, and neuronal pathways, have been proposed in this bidirectional communication between the immune system and the brain after surgery.

Notably, strategies aimed at mitigating the excessive inflammatory milieu have been promising in limiting surgery-induced cognitive decline in several rodent models and may offer novel insights for future interventional studies in humans.

Ongoing clinical studies are starting to uncover a potential role for blood and cerebrospinal fluid (CSF) inflammatory biomarkers in the pathophysiology of POCD, and this represents a burgeoning area of research for the field. However, it remains unclear to what extent the findings in animal models translate to human patients. Although mice are useful for modeling spatial memory deficits after anesthesia and surgery, mice lack the ability to perform more complex human cognitive functions, such as executive function. Thus, mouse models may be useful for understanding some of the memory deficits seen in human POCD, but they cannot recapitulate the full spectrum of cognitive deficits seen in our patients. Also, it is challenging to model the temporal course of human POCD in rodents: preclinical studies often report acute cognitive changes in hippocampal-dependent cognitive tasks but provide limited evidence for longer-lasting neurocognitive dysfunction. Combining anesthesia/surgical trauma with known risk factors for POCD (ie, aging, infection, metabolic syndrome) in rodents may provide a more relevant model of human POCD.[87–89] Further, given the significant differences between the mouse and human immune systems and inflammatory mechanisms,[90] it is unclear to what extent the neuroinflammatory mechanisms seen in mouse models are involved in human POCD.

One recent animal study also suggested that postoperative memory deficits may be due to anesthetic-induced upregulation of alpha-5 subunit containing gamma-aminobutyric acid (GABA)-A receptors in the hippocampus.[91] These alpha-5–containing GABA receptors inhibit long-term potentiation (LTP, a cellular correlate of learning and memory). Thus, upregulation of these receptors would be predicted to cause learning and memory deficits, which could play a role in contributing to human POCD and/or postoperative delirium. However, it is unclear whether anesthetic drugs and/or inflammatory mediators that impinge on LTP function also cause a sustained upregulation of alpha-5 GABA-A receptors in humans.

Human Studies

The mouse studies described previously provide useful hypotheses about what might cause POCD, which can then be investigated in human studies. Indeed, surgery is associated with a central neuroinflammatory response in humans.[92–96] It remains unclear, though, whether this central neuroinflammatory response is associated with POCD. To the best of our knowledge, no human studies have demonstrated an association between the presence or levels of central inflammatory mediators and the presence or duration of POCD. Preexisting AD pathology (as measured by CSF biomarkers) has been associated with increased perioperative decline in some cognitive tests but not in others,[97] and patients with MCI, a prodromal stage of AD, have larger cognitive deficits in some tests after perioperative care than surgical patients without MCI.[98,99] These studies suggest that preexisting AD pathology may be associated with POCD, but the full extent of this relationship remains to be elucidated. One recent pilot study also found that the extent of preexisting white matter damage (as measured by MRI) was a predictor of postoperative executive function deficits in patients who underwent knee arthroplasty.[100] Neuroimaging studies also have shown that cardiac surgery in particular is associated with an increase in "silent strokes" or white matter hyperintensities seen on MRI, although the total burden of white matter hyperintensities after surgery does not correlate with the presence of POCD[101,102] (reviewed in Ref.[32]). Clearly, understanding the relationship between central neuroinflammation, cerebrovascular white matter disease, AD pathology (and/or perioperative changes in these processes) and POCD is a major question in the field.

Numerous human studies have failed to find plasma biomarkers associated with POCD,[11,103] although one recent study found that higher plasma levels of copeptin (a peptide co-released with arginine vasopressin from the hypothalamus) were associated with increased risk of both postoperative delirium and POCD.[104] Remarkably, plasma copeptin levels were a better predictor of POCD risk than age in this study[104]; it will be important to replicate these results. The failure of numerous other studies to find plasma biomarkers of POCD may be due to differential protein and cytokine expression between the cerebrospinal fluid and plasma.[94] Future human studies combining CSF biomarker measurements, cognitive testing, and functional neuroimaging both before and after perioperative care will be necessary to further elucidate the pathophysiology of POCD, and to fully ascertain whether anesthesia and surgery are associated with an acceleration of AD pathology.[28,105]

HOW CAN WE PREVENT OR TREAT POSTOPERATIVE COGNITIVE DYSFUNCTION?
Postoperative Cognitive Dysfunction Prevention Studies

Although we are likely only in the infancy of understanding the etiologies of POCD, its detrimental impact on patients mandate that clinicians do everything in their power to prevent patients from developing POCD and to treat POCD once it does develop. Numerous investigators have attempted to prevent POCD with interventions ranging from intraoperative lidocaine,[66] magnesium,[106] ketamine,[107] complement suppression,[108] or even high-dose dexamethasone[109] treatment in randomized controlled trials. Lidocaine treatment had no effect on preventing POCD overall,[66] although in a secondary analysis, lidocaine infusion appeared to have a beneficial effect on cognition in nondiabetic patients. Similarly, intraoperative magnesium treatment had no effect on preventing POCD overall, although there was a trend toward a detrimental effect of magnesium treatment on cognition in heavier patients.[106] Complement suppression with the monoclonal antibody pexelizumab (which inhibits complement factor C5) also had no effect on the rate of POCD, although it was associated with improved visuospatial cognition.[108]

Surprisingly, ketamine treatment (0.5 mg/kg) on anesthetic induction was associated with a decrease in POCD occurrence after cardiac surgery.[107] Ketamine treatment also was associated with a reduction in serum C-reactive protein levels in this study,[107] leading the investigators to propose that ketamine decreases POCD incidence by decreasing inflammation. However, high-dose dexamethasone (ie, 1 mg/kg on anesthetic induction) did not decrease POCD rates in patients undergoing cardiac surgery in the Dexamethasone for Cardiac Surgery (DECS) trial,[109] which was almost 4 times the size of the ketamine trial.[107] Higher-dose dexamethasone (0.2 mg/kg) was actually associated with increased POCD rates (as compared with 0.1 mg/kg dexamethasone or placebo treatment) in a trial of patients undergoing microvascular decompression for facial spasms.[110] Taken together, these results could imply that although inflammation may play a role in POCD, not all drugs with anti-inflammatory activity have the same effects on POCD. Alternatively, the efficacy of ketamine in reducing POCD[107] may be due to its effects on neurotransmitter receptors or other biological processes unrelated to inflammation; in addition to blocking the N-methyl-D-aspartate receptor, ketamine modulates signaling via a number of other receptors (reviewed in Ref.[111]).

Although the failure of numerous single-drug therapies for POCD prevention are disappointing, these failures are not surprising if POCD is viewed as a syndrome of brain dysfunction caused by diverse factors rather than a single disease caused by a specific etiology. Further, the complexity of the human brain itself is staggering: it contains more than 80 billion neurons (each of which make thousands of synaptic connections to other neurons), and more than 80 billion interneurons.[112] The human brain also expresses more than 80% of the human genome,[113] a higher percentage than any other organ. Considering the complexity of the human brain, and the diverse factors that may contribute to POCD, it is less surprising that several single-drug interventions failed to reduce the incidence of POCD.

Preventing POCD may thus require a multicomponent intervention that addresses the diverse factors that contribute to its genesis. A recent pilot study suggested that remote ischemic preconditioning may decrease cognitive deficits after cardiac surgery.[114] Because remote ischemic preconditioning has a plethora of biological effects,[115] this study is consistent with the idea that preventing POCD will require interventions that work more broadly than a single drug.

Similarly, Ballard and colleagues[24] examined the effect of a combined intervention to decrease POCD rates, which included intraoperative bispectral index monitoring (to optimally titrate anesthetic depth) and cerebral oxygen saturation monitoring (to titrate cerebral oxygen delivery). This combined intervention reduced POCD incidence at multiple time points (see **Table 2** for statistics). However, there is mixed evidence whether bispectral (BIS) index monitoring alone can decrease POCD rates,[51,52] and the investigators of a systematic review also concluded that there is insufficient evidence to recommend the use of cerebral oximetry monitoring on its own to decrease POCD rates after cardiac surgery.[116] Taken together, these studies may mean that the combined use of BIS and cerebral oximetry monitoring may help decrease POCD rates, but that either monitor alone may have a lesser or nonsignificant effect. Future studies will be necessary to examine this hypothesis by evaluating these interventions in isolation and together.

Postoperative Cognitive Dysfunction Treatment Studies

Very few randomized controlled studies have examined whether any intervention can treat or improve POCD once it has already occurred. Such studies are challenging to conduct, as most cases of POCD resolve spontaneously within months (see the section "A description of postoperative cognitive dysfunction and postoperative cognitive improvement"), although they would still be important given the association between POCD and decreased quality of life,[18] early exit from the workforce,[19] and premature mortality.[19,20] However, these studies would be neither unprecedented nor impossible; a similar challenge occurs in depression treatment trials, in which there is a high response even among patients receiving placebo within weeks to months.[117] One randomized trial examined the use of the acetylcholinesterase inhibitor donepezil in patients who displayed cognitive decline (0.5 SD drop in at least 1 cognitive domain) 1 year after cardiac surgery. Donepezil improved some aspects of memory performance in these patients, which is consistent with the role of acetylcholinesterase inhibitors in improving memory in patients with early-stage AD. However, donepezil treatment had no effect on the overall cognitive index in these patients with cognitive decline 1 year after cardiac surgery.[118]

Interestingly, the antidepressant and selective serotonin reuptake inhibitor (SSRI) citalopram was used to successfully treat POCD in one case report.[119] This finding is generally in line with the pleiotropic biological roles of serotonin, including its ability to promote neuroplasticity.[120] If POCD is a syndrome of failed resilience or a lack of neuroplasticity after perioperative care that occurs in patients with preexisting neurovascular disease or "silent strokes," then the established efficacy of SSRIs in improving neurologic outcomes after stroke[121] suggests that they may be useful in treating POCD as well. SSRIs also have been shown to improve quality of life in depressed elderly patients[122] and improve affect and mood even in nondepressed, healthy individuals,[123] which further suggests that SSRIs may be efficacious in reducing POCD-associated quality-of-life impairments. More work will be necessary to determine whether SSRIs improve cognition, quality of life, and other outcomes in patients with POCD (see **Table 4**).

SUMMARY AND FUTURE DIRECTIONS

POCD is a syndrome that occurs more frequently in patients age 60 and older, and is associated with early exit from the workforce,[19] decreased quality of life,[18] and premature mortality.[19,20] It typically lasts for weeks to months,[23] although rare cases may last considerably longer.[1] Based on this understanding, we believe that patients at high risk for POCD (ie, those with multiple risk factors listed in **Tables 2** and **3**, such as elderly patients) should be counseled preoperatively about the risk of POCD, just as we counsel patients preoperatively about numerous other risks of perioperative care. This counseling could allow patients to make cognitively demanding decisions before surgery/anesthesia, and/or to ensure that they will have loved ones or others to help them with cognitively demanding tasks for the first weeks to months after surgery/anesthesia. Additional help and assistance may help these patients recover better from surgery in general; after all, patients with POCD who may not be able to remember what they ate for breakfast that morning are also unlikely to be able to remember whether they took their medicine that morning.

The long-term sequelae of POCD also mandates that we try to prevent it, and that we develop effect treatments for it once it has occurred. The failure of numerous intervention trials to prevent POCD, and our general lack of understanding of what causes POCD, argue that developing a better understanding of the etiology of POCD may be essential for developing strategies to prevent it. We have conceptualized POCD as a failure of resilience in the face of perioperative stress, which suggests that strategies to improve physical and cognitive resilience in the elderly may help prevent POCD and improve overall recovery after surgery.

ACKNOWLEDGEMENTS

Dr M. Berger acknowledges grant funding from the International Anesthesia Research Society (Mentored Research Award) and the National Institute of Health (T32 #GM08600). Dr J. Browndyke acknowledges funding from the following grants: NIA R01-AG042599, NHLBI R01-HL109219, and NHLBI R21-HL109971. Dr H. Whitson acknowledges funding from the following grants: NIH R01AG043438, NIH R24AG045050, Alzheimer's Association NIRG-13-282202, and VA I21 RX001721-01. Dr Whitson's and Cohen's contributions are supported by Duke Pepper Center (P30AG028716). Dr J. Mathew acknowledges support from NIH grants HL096978, HL108280, and HL109971.

REFERENCES

1. Bedford PD. Adverse cerebral effects of anaesthesia on old people. Lancet 1955;269:259–63.
2. Fontes MT, Swift RC, Phillips-Bute B, et al, Neurologic Outcome Research Group of the Duke Heart Center. Predictors of cognitive recovery after cardiac surgery. Anesth Analg 2013;116:435–42.

3. Alosco ML, Galioto R, Spitznagel MB, et al. Cognitive function after bariatric surgery: evidence for improvement 3 years after surgery. Am J Surg 2014;207: 870–6.
4. Alosco ML, Spitznagel MB, Strain G, et al. Improved memory function two years after bariatric surgery. Obesity (Silver Spring) 2014;22:32–8.
5. Weiser TG, Regenbogen SE, Thompson KD, et al. An estimation of the global volume of surgery: a modelling strategy based on available data. Lancet 2008;372:139–44.
6. Kapur S, Phillips AG, Insel TR. Why has it taken so long for biological psychiatry to develop clinical tests and what to do about it? Mol Psychiatry 2012;17: 1174–9.
7. Newman MF, Kirchner JL, Phillips-Bute B, et al. Longitudinal assessment of neurocognitive function after coronary-artery bypass surgery. N Engl J Med 2001; 344:395–402.
8. Selnes OA, Grega MA, Bailey MM, et al. Do management strategies for coronary artery disease influence 6-year cognitive outcomes? Ann Thorac Surg 2009;88: 445–54.
9. Saczynski JS, Marcantonio ER, Quach L, et al. Cognitive trajectories after postoperative delirium. N Engl J Med 2012;367:30–9.
10. Funder KS, Steinmetz J, Rasmussen LS. Methodological issues of postoperative cognitive dysfunction research. Semin Cardiothorac Vasc Anesth 2010;14: 119–22.
11. McDonagh DL, Mathew JP, White WD, et al. Cognitive function after major noncardiac surgery, apolipoprotein E4 genotype, and biomarkers of brain injury. Anesthesiology 2010;112:852–9.
12. Avidan MS, Xiong C, Evers AS. Postoperative cognitive decline: the unsubstantiated phenotype. Anesthesiology 2010;113:1246–8 [author reply: 1248–50].
13. Levine AJ, Miller EN, Becker JT, et al. Normative data for determining significance of test-retest differences on eight common neuropsychological instruments. Clin Neuropsychol 2004;18:373–84.
14. Duff K. Evidence-based indicators of neuropsychological change in the individual patient: relevant concepts and methods. Arch Clin Neuropsychol 2012;27: 248–61.
15. Jacobson NS, Truax P. Clinical significance: a statistical approach to defining meaningful change in psychotherapy research. J Consult Clin Psychol 1991; 59:12–9.
16. Lewis MS, Maruff P, Silbert BS, et al. The sensitivity and specificity of three common statistical rules for the classification of post-operative cognitive dysfunction following coronary artery bypass graft surgery. Acta Anaesthesiol Scand 2006; 50:50–7.
17. Petersen RC. Mild cognitive impairment as a diagnostic entity. J Intern Med 2004;256:183–94.
18. Phillips-Bute B, Mathew JP, Blumenthal JA, et al. Association of neurocognitive function and quality of life 1 year after coronary artery bypass graft (CABG) surgery. Psychosom Med 2006;68:369–75.
19. Steinmetz J, Christensen KB, Lund T, et al. Long-term consequences of postoperative cognitive dysfunction. Anesthesiology 2009;110:548–55.
20. Monk TG, Weldon BC, Garvan CW, et al. Predictors of cognitive dysfunction after major noncardiac surgery. Anesthesiology 2008;108:18–30.
21. Nadelson MR, Sanders RD, Avidan MS. Perioperative cognitive trajectory in adults. Br J Anaesth 2014;112:440–51.

22. Avidan MS, Evers AS. Review of clinical evidence for persistent cognitive decline or incident dementia attributable to surgery or general anesthesia. J Alzheimers Dis 2011;24:201–16.

23. Moller JT, Cluitmans P, Rasmussen LS, et al. Long-term postoperative cognitive dysfunction in the elderly ISPOCD1 study. ISPOCD investigators. International Study of Post-Operative Cognitive Dysfunction. Lancet 1998;351:857–61.

24. Ballard C, Jones E, Gauge N, et al. Optimised anaesthesia to reduce post operative cognitive decline (POCD) in older patients undergoing elective surgery, a randomised controlled trial. PLoS One 2012;7:e37410.

25. Avidan MS, Searleman AC, Storandt M, et al. Long-term cognitive decline in older subjects was not attributable to noncardiac surgery or major illness. Anesthesiology 2009;111:964–70.

26. Chen PL, Yang CW, Tseng YK, et al. Risk of dementia after anaesthesia and surgery. Br J Psychiatry 2014;204:188–93.

27. Chen CW, Lin CC, Chen KB, et al. Increased risk of dementia in people with previous exposure to general anesthesia: a nationwide population-based case-control study. Alzheimers Dement 2014;10:196–204.

28. Berger M, Burke J, Eckenhoff R, et al. Alzheimer's disease, anesthesia, and surgery: a clinically focused review. J Cardiothorac Vasc Anesth 2014;28:1609–23.

29. Selnes OA, Grega MA, Bailey MM, et al. Cognition 6 years after surgical or medical therapy for coronary artery disease. Ann Neurol 2008;63:581–90.

30. Selnes OA, Grega MA, Bailey MM, et al. Neurocognitive outcomes 3 years after coronary artery bypass graft surgery: a controlled study. Ann Thorac Surg 2007; 84:1885–96.

31. Sauer AM, Nathoe HM, Hendrikse J, et al, Octopus Study Group. Cognitive outcomes 7.5 years after angioplasty compared with off-pump coronary bypass surgery. Ann Thorac Surg 2013;96:1294–300.

32. McDonagh DL, Berger M, Mathew JP, et al. Neurological complications of cardiac surgery. Lancet Neurol 2014;13:490–502.

33. Bartels K, McDonagh DL, Newman MF, et al. Neurocognitive outcomes after cardiac surgery. Curr Opin Anaesthesiol 2013;26:91–7.

34. Evered L, Scott DA, Silbert B, et al. Postoperative cognitive dysfunction is independent of type of surgery and anesthetic. Anesth Analg 2011;112:1179–85.

35. Hemmingsen R, Mejsholm B, Vorstrup S, et al. Carotid surgery, cognitive function, and cerebral blood flow in patients with transient ischemic attacks. Ann Neurol 1986;20:13–9.

36. Raeder MB, Helland CA, Hugdahl K, et al. Arachnoid cysts cause cognitive deficits that improve after surgery. Neurology 2005;64:160–2.

37. Casey JE, Ferguson GG, Kimura D, et al. Neuropsychological improvement versus practice effect following unilateral carotid endarterectomy in patients without stroke. J Clin Exp Neuropsychol 1989;11:461–70.

38. Rasmussen LS, Siersma VD, Ispocd G. Postoperative cognitive dysfunction: true deterioration versus random variation. Acta Anaesthesiol Scand 2004;48: 1137–43.

39. Cormack F, Shipolini A, Awad WI, et al. A meta-analysis of cognitive outcome following coronary artery bypass graft surgery. Neurosci Biobehav Rev 2012; 36:2118–29.

40. Lindquist R, Dupuis G, Terrin ML, et al, POST CABG Biobehavioral Study Investigators. Comparison of health-related quality-of-life outcomes of men and women after coronary artery bypass surgery through 1 year: findings from the POST CABG Biobehavioral Study. Am Heart J 2003;146:1038–44.

41. Rabbitt P, Donlan C, Watson P, et al. Unique and interactive effects of depression, age, socioeconomic advantage, and gender on cognitive performance of normal healthy older people. Psychol Aging 1995;10:307–13.
42. Norman S, Troster AI, Fields JA, et al. Effects of depression and Parkinson's disease on cognitive functioning. J Neuropsychiatry Clin Neurosci 2002;14:31–6.
43. Janelsins MC, Kesler SR, Ahles TA, et al. Prevalence, mechanisms, and management of cancer-related cognitive impairment. Int Rev Psychiatry 2014;26:102–13.
44. Saykin AJ, Ahles TA, McDonald BC. Mechanisms of chemotherapy-induced cognitive disorders: neuropsychological, pathophysiological, and neuroimaging perspectives. Semin Clin Neuropsychiatry 2003;8:201–16.
45. Maier SF, Watkins LR. Immune-to-central nervous system communication and its role in modulating pain and cognition: implications for cancer and cancer treatment. Brain Behav Immun 2003;17(Suppl 1):S125–31.
46. Ahles TA, Saykin AJ, McDonald BC, et al. Longitudinal assessment of cognitive changes associated with adjuvant treatment for breast cancer: impact of age and cognitive reserve. J Clin Oncol 2010;28:4434–40.
47. Schilder CM, Seynaeve C, Beex LV, et al. Effects of tamoxifen and exemestane on cognitive functioning of postmenopausal patients with breast cancer: results from the neuropsychological side study of the tamoxifen and exemestane adjuvant multinational trial. J Clin Oncol 2010;28:1294–300.
48. Falleti MG, Sanfilippo A, Maruff P, et al. The nature and severity of cognitive impairment associated with adjuvant chemotherapy in women with breast cancer: a meta-analysis of the current literature. Brain Cogn 2005;59:60–70.
49. Johnson T, Monk T, Rasmussen LS, et al, ISPOCD2 Investigators. Postoperative cognitive dysfunction in middle-aged patients. Anesthesiology 2002;96:1351–7.
50. Correa DD, Hess LM. Cognitive function and quality of life in ovarian cancer. Gynecol Oncol 2012;124:404–9.
51. Chan MT, Cheng BC, Lee TM, et al. BIS-guided anesthesia decreases postoperative delirium and cognitive decline. J Neurosurg Anesthesiol 2013;25:33–42.
52. Radtke FM, Franck M, Lendner J, et al. Monitoring depth of anaesthesia in a randomized trial decreases the rate of postoperative delirium but not postoperative cognitive dysfunction. Br J Anaesth 2013;110(Suppl 1):i98–105.
53. Rasmussen LS, Johnson T, Kuipers HM, et al, ISPOCD2 Investigators. Does anaesthesia cause postoperative cognitive dysfunction? A randomised study of regional versus general anaesthesia in 438 elderly patients. Acta Anaesthesiol Scand 2003;47:260–6.
54. Silbert BS, Evered LA, Scott DA. Incidence of postoperative cognitive dysfunction after general or spinal anaesthesia for extracorporeal shock wave lithotripsy. Br J Anaesth 2014;113:784–91.
55. Mason SE, Noel-Storr A, Ritchie CW. The impact of general and regional anesthesia on the incidence of post-operative cognitive dysfunction and postoperative delirium: a systematic review with meta-analysis. J Alzheimers Dis 2010;22(Suppl 3):67–79.
56. Guay J. General anaesthesia does not contribute to long-term post-operative cognitive dysfunction in adults: a meta-analysis. Indian J Anaesth 2011;55: 358–63.
57. Cai Y, Hu H, Liu P, et al. Association between the apolipoprotein E4 and postoperative cognitive dysfunction in elderly patients undergoing intravenous anesthesia and inhalation anesthesia. Anesthesiology 2012;116:84–93.
58. Deiner S, Baxter MG. Cognitive dysfunction after inhalation versus intravenous anesthesia in elderly patients. Anesthesiology 2012;117:676–8 [author reply: 8].

59. Rortgen D, Kloos J, Fries M, et al. Comparison of early cognitive function and recovery after desflurane or sevoflurane anaesthesia in the elderly: a double-blinded randomized controlled trial. Br J Anaesth 2010;104:167–74.
60. Zhang B, Tian M, Zhen Y, et al. The effects of isoflurane and desflurane on cognitive function in humans. Anesth Analg 2012;114:410–5.
61. Kanbak M, Saricaoglu F, Akinci SB, et al. The effects of isoflurane, sevoflurane, and desflurane anesthesia on neurocognitive outcome after cardiac surgery: a pilot study. Heart Surg Forum 2007;10:E36–41.
62. Schoen J, Husemann L, Tiemeyer C, et al. Cognitive function after sevoflurane-vs propofol-based anaesthesia for on-pump cardiac surgery: a randomized controlled trial. Br J Anaesth 2011;106:840–50.
63. Liu Y, Pan N, Ma Y, et al. Inhaled sevoflurane may promote progression of amnestic mild cognitive impairment: a prospective, randomized parallel-group study. Am J Med Sci 2013;345:355–60.
64. Tang N, Ou C, Liu Y, et al. Effect of inhalational anaesthetic on postoperative cognitive dysfunction following radical rectal resection in elderly patients with mild cognitive impairment. J Int Med Res 2014;42:1252–61.
65. Griebe M, Amann M, Hirsch JG, et al. Reduced functional reserve in patients with age-related white matter changes: a preliminary FMRI study of working memory. PLoS One 2014;9:e103359.
66. Mathew JP, Mackensen GB, Phillips-Bute B, et al, Neurologic Outcome Research Group of the Duke Heart Center. Randomized, double-blinded, placebo controlled study of neuroprotection with lidocaine in cardiac surgery. Stroke 2009;40:880–7.
67. Mathew JP, Podgoreanu MV, Grocott HP, et al, PEGASUS Investigative Team. Genetic variants in P-selectin and C-reactive protein influence susceptibility to cognitive decline after cardiac surgery. J Am Coll Cardiol 2007;49:1934–42.
68. Brown M, Sinacore DR, Ehsani AA, et al. Low-intensity exercise as a modifier of physical frailty in older adults. Arch Phys Med Rehabil 2000;81:960–5.
69. Binder EF, Schechtman KB, Ehsani AA, et al. Effects of exercise training on frailty in community-dwelling older adults: results of a randomized, controlled trial. J Am Geriatr Soc 2002;50:1921–8.
70. Mohandas A, Reifsnyder J, Jacobs M, et al. Current and future directions in frailty research. Popul Health Manag 2011;14:277–83.
71. Cameron ID, Fairhall N, Langron C, et al. A multifactorial interdisciplinary intervention reduces frailty in older people: randomized trial. BMC Med 2013;11:65.
72. Gillis C, Li C, Lee L, et al. Prehabilitation versus rehabilitation: a randomized control trial in patients undergoing colorectal resection for cancer. Anesthesiology 2014;121:937–47.
73. Jaggers JR, Simpson CD, Frost KL, et al. Prehabilitation before knee arthroplasty increases postsurgical function: a case study. J Strength Cond Res 2007;21:632–4.
74. Nielsen PR, Andreasen J, Asmussen M, et al. Costs and quality of life for prehabilitation and early rehabilitation after surgery of the lumbar spine. BMC Health Serv Res 2008;8:209.
75. Furze G, Dumville JC, Miles JN, et al. "Prehabilitation" prior to CABG surgery improves physical functioning and depression. Int J Cardiol 2009;132:51–8.
76. Erickson KI, Voss MW, Prakash RS, et al. Exercise training increases size of hippocampus and improves memory. Proc Natl Acad Sci U S A 2011;108: 3017–22.

77. Maguire EA, Gadian DG, Johnsrude IS, et al. Navigation-related structural change in the hippocampi of taxi drivers. Proc Natl Acad Sci U S A 2000;97: 4398–403.
78. Burke SN, Barnes CA. Neural plasticity in the ageing brain. Nat Rev Neurosci 2006;7:30–40.
79. Terrando N, Monaco C, Ma D, et al. Tumor necrosis factor-alpha triggers a cytokine cascade yielding postoperative cognitive decline. Proc Natl Acad Sci U S A 2010;107:20518–22.
80. Terrando N, Eriksson LI, Ryu JK, et al. Resolving postoperative neuroinflammation and cognitive decline. Ann Neurol 2011;70:986–95.
81. Su X, Feng X, Terrando N, et al. Dysfunction of inflammation-resolving pathways is associated with exaggerated postoperative cognitive decline in a rat model of the metabolic syndrome. Mol Med 2012;18:1481–90.
82. Bartels K, Ma Q, Venkatraman TN, et al. Effects of deep hypothermic circulatory arrest on the blood brain barrier in a cardiopulmonary bypass model–a pilot study. Heart Lung Circ 2014;23:981–4.
83. Hu N, Guo D, Wang H, et al. Involvement of the blood-brain barrier opening in cognitive decline in aged rats following orthopedic surgery and high concentration of sevoflurane inhalation. Brain Res 2014;1551:13–24.
84. He HJ, Wang Y, Le Y, et al. Surgery upregulates high mobility group box-1 and disrupts the blood-brain barrier causing cognitive dysfunction in aged rats. CNS Neurosci Ther 2012;18:994–1002.
85. Degos V, Vacas S, Han Z, et al. Depletion of bone marrow-derived macrophages perturbs the innate immune response to surgery and reduces postoperative memory dysfunction. Anesthesiology 2013;118:527–36.
86. Vacas S, Degos V, Tracey KJ, et al. High-mobility group box 1 protein initiates postoperative cognitive decline by engaging bone marrow-derived macrophages. Anesthesiology 2014;120:1160–7.
87. Rosczyk HA, Sparkman NL, Johnson RW. Neuroinflammation and cognitive function in aged mice following minor surgery. Exp Gerontol 2008;43:840–6.
88. Terrando N, Yang T, Ryu JK, et al. Stimulation of the alpha 7 nicotinic acetylcholine receptor protects against neuroinflammation after tibia fracture and endotoxemia in mice. Mol Med 2015;20(1):667–75.
89. Feng X, Degos V, Koch LG, et al. Surgery results in exaggerated and persistent cognitive decline in a rat model of the metabolic syndrome. Anesthesiology 2013;118:1098–105.
90. Zschaler J, Schlorke D, Arnhold J. Differences in innate immune response between man and mouse. Crit Rev Immunol 2014;34:433–54.
91. Zurek AA, Yu J, Wang DS, et al. Sustained increase in alpha5GABAA receptor function impairs memory after anesthesia. J Clin Invest 2014;124:5437–41.
92. Yeager MP, Lunt P, Arruda J, et al. Cerebrospinal fluid cytokine levels after surgery with spinal or general anesthesia. Reg Anesth Pain Med 1999;24: 557–62.
93. Tang JX, Baranov D, Hammond M, et al. Human Alzheimer and inflammation biomarkers after anesthesia and surgery. Anesthesiology 2011;115:727–32.
94. Buvanendran A, Kroin JS, Berger RA, et al. Upregulation of prostaglandin E2 and interleukins in the central nervous system and peripheral tissue during and after surgery in humans. Anesthesiology 2006;104:403–10.
95. Reis HJ, Teixeira AL, Kalman J, et al. Different inflammatory biomarker patterns in the cerebro-spinal fluid following heart surgery and major non-cardiac operations. Curr Drug Metab 2007;8:639–42.

96. Reinsfelt B, Westerlind A, Blennow K, et al. Open-heart surgery increases cerebrospinal fluid levels of Alzheimer-associated amyloid beta. Acta Anaesthesiol Scand 2013;57:82–8.
97. Xie Z, McAuliffe S, Swain CA, et al. Cerebrospinal fluid: a beta to tau ratio and postoperative cognitive change. Ann Surg 2013;258:364–9.
98. Kline RP, Pirraglia E, Cheng H, et al. Surgery and brain atrophy in cognitively normal elderly subjects and subjects diagnosed with mild cognitive impairment. Anesthesiology 2012;116:603–12.
99. Bekker A, Lee C, de Santi S, et al. Does mild cognitive impairment increase the risk of developing postoperative cognitive dysfunction? Am J Surg 2010;199: 782–8.
100. Price CC, Tanner JJ, Schmalfuss I, et al. A pilot study evaluating presurgery neuroanatomical biomarkers for postoperative cognitive decline after total knee arthroplasty in older adults. Anesthesiology 2014;120:601–13.
101. Cook DJ, Huston J 3rd, Trenerry MR, et al. Postcardiac surgical cognitive impairment in the aged using diffusion-weighted magnetic resonance imaging. Ann Thorac Surg 2007;83:1389–95.
102. Rodriguez RA, Rubens FD, Wozny D, et al. Cerebral emboli detected by transcranial Doppler during cardiopulmonary bypass are not correlated with postoperative cognitive deficits. Stroke 2010;41:2229–35.
103. Gerriets T, Schwarz N, Bachmann G, et al. Evaluation of methods to predict early long-term neurobehavioral outcome after coronary artery bypass grafting. Am J Cardiol 2010;105:1095–101.
104. Dong S, Li CL, Liang WD, et al. Postoperative plasma copeptin levels independently predict delirium and cognitive dysfunction after coronary artery bypass graft surgery. Peptides 2014;59:70–4.
105. Terrando N, Eriksson LI, Eckenhoff RG. Perioperative neurotoxicity in the elderly: summary of the 4th international workshop. Anesth Analg 2015;120:649–52.
106. Mathew JP, White WD, Schinderle DB, et al, Neurologic Outcome Research Group of the Duke Heart Center. Intraoperative magnesium administration does not improve neurocognitive function after cardiac surgery. Stroke 2013; 44:3407–13.
107. Hudetz JA, Iqbal Z, Gandhi SD, et al. Ketamine attenuates post-operative cognitive dysfunction after cardiac surgery. Acta Anaesthesiol Scand 2009;53:864–72.
108. Mathew JP, Shernan SK, White WD, et al. Preliminary report of the effects of complement suppression with pexelizumab on neurocognitive decline after coronary artery bypass graft surgery. Stroke 2004;35:2335–9.
109. Ottens TH, Dieleman JM, Sauer AM, et al, DExamethasone for Cardiac Surgery (DECS) Study Group. Effects of dexamethasone on cognitive decline after cardiac surgery: a randomized clinical trial. Anesthesiology 2014;121:492–500.
110. Fang Q, Qian X, An J, et al. Higher dose dexamethasone increases early postoperative cognitive dysfunction. J Neurosurg Anesthesiol 2014;26:220–5.
111. Potter DE, Choudhury M. Ketamine: repurposing and redefining a multifaceted drug. Drug Discov Today 2014;19:1848–54.
112. Azevedo FA, Carvalho LR, Grinberg LT, et al. Equal numbers of neuronal and nonneuronal cells make the human brain an isometrically scaled-up primate brain. J Comp Neurol 2009;513:532–41.
113. Hawrylycz MJ, Lein ES, Guillozet-Bongaarts AL, et al. An anatomically comprehensive atlas of the adult human brain transcriptome. Nature 2012;489:391–9.
114. Hudetz JA, Patterson KM, Iqbal Z, et al. Remote ischemic preconditioning prevents deterioration of short-term postoperative cognitive function after cardiac

surgery using cardiopulmonary bypass: results of a pilot investigation. J Cardiothorac Vasc Anesth 2015;29(2):382–8.

115. Gill R, Kuriakose R, Gertz ZM, et al. Remote ischemic preconditioning for myocardial protection: update on mechanisms and clinical relevance. Mol Cell Biochem 2015;402(1–2):41–9.

116. Zheng F, Sheinberg R, Yee MS, et al. Cerebral near-infrared spectroscopy monitoring and neurologic outcomes in adult cardiac surgery patients: a systematic review. Anesth Analg 2013;116:663–76.

117. Keller M, Montgomery S, Ball W, et al. Lack of efficacy of the substance p (neurokinin1 receptor) antagonist aprepitant in the treatment of major depressive disorder. Biol Psychiatry 2006;59:216–23.

118. Doraiswamy PM, Babyak MA, Hennig T, et al. Donepezil for cognitive decline following coronary artery bypass surgery: a pilot randomized controlled trial. Psychopharmacol Bull 2007;40:54–62.

119. Yap KK, Joyner P. Post-operative cognitive dysfunction after knee arthroplasty: a diagnostic dilemma. Oxf Med Case Reports 2014;3:60–2.

120. Berger M, Gray JA, Roth BL. The expanded biology of serotonin. Annu Rev Med 2009;60:355–66.

121. Chollet F, Tardy J, Albucher JF, et al. Fluoxetine for motor recovery after acute ischaemic stroke (FLAME): a randomised placebo-controlled trial. Lancet Neurol 2011;10:123–30.

122. Heiligenstein JH, Ware JE Jr, Beusterien KM, et al. Acute effects of fluoxetine versus placebo on functional health and well-being in late-life depression. Int Psychogeriatr 1995;7(Suppl):125–37.

123. Knutson B, Wolkowitz OM, Cole SW, et al. Selective alteration of personality and social behavior by serotonergic intervention. Am J Psychiatry 1998;155:373–9.

124. Hewitt J, Williams M, Pearce L, et al. The prevalence of cognitive impairment in emergency general surgery. Int J Surg 2014;12:1031–5.

125. Nasreddine ZS, Phillips NA, Bedirian V, et al. The Montreal Cognitive Assessment, MoCA: a brief screening tool for mild cognitive impairment. J Am Geriatr Soc 2005;53:695–9.

126. Aleman A, van't Wout M. Repetitive transcranial magnetic stimulation over the right dorsolateral prefrontal cortex disrupts digit span task performance. Neuropsychobiology 2008;57:44–8.

127. Hudetz JA, Patterson KM, Amole O, et al. Postoperative cognitive dysfunction after noncardiac surgery: effects of metabolic syndrome. J Anesth 2011;25:337–44.

128. Takeuchi H, Taki Y, Sassa Y, et al. Regional gray and white matter volume associated with Stroop interference: evidence from voxel-based morphometry. Neuroimage 2012;59:2899–907.

129. Vazzana R, Bandinelli S, Lauretani F, et al. Trail making test predicts physical impairment and mortality in older persons. J Am Geriatr Soc 2010;58:719–23.

130. Oosterman JM, Vogels RL, van Harten B, et al. Assessing mental flexibility: neuroanatomical and neuropsychological correlates of the trail making test in elderly people. Clin Neuropsychol 2010;24:203–19.

131. Audenaert K, Brans B, Van Laere K, et al. Verbal fluency as a prefrontal activation probe: a validation study using 99mTc-ECD brain SPET. Eur J Nucl Med 2000;27:1800–8.

132. Wood AG, Saling MM, Abbott DF, et al. A neurocognitive account of frontal lobe involvement in orthographic lexical retrieval: an fMRI study. Neuroimage 2001;14:162–9.

133. Strangman GE, O'Neil-Pirozzi TM, Goldstein R, et al. Prediction of memory reha-bilitation outcomes in traumatic brain injury by using functional magnetic reso-nance imaging. Arch Phys Med Rehabil 2008;89:974–81.
134. Kane KD, Yochim BP. Construct validity and extended normative data for older adults for the brief visuospatial memory test, revised. Am J Alzheimers Dis Other Demen 2014;29:601–6.
135. Gawryluk JR, Mazerolle EL, Beyea SD, et al. Functional MRI activation in white matter during the symbol digit modalities test. Front Hum Neurosci 2014;8:589.
136. Forn C, Rocca MA, Bosca I, et al. Analysis of "task-positive" and "task-negative" functional networks during the performance of the symbol digit modalities test in patients at presentation with clinically isolated syndrome suggestive of multiple sclerosis. Exp Brain Res 2013;225:399–407.
137. Moritz CH, Johnson SC, McMillan KM, et al. Functional MRI neuroanatomic cor-relates of the Hooper Visual Organization Test. J Int Neuropsychol Soc 2004;10: 939–47.
138. Bohnen NI, Kuwabara H, Constantine GM, et al. Grooved pegboard test as a biomarker of nigrostriatal denervation in Parkinson's disease. Neurosci Lett 2007;424:185–9.
139. Logothetis NK. What we can do and what we cannot do with fMRI. Nature 2008; 453:869–78.
140. Ropper AH. Cogito ergo sum by MRI. N Engl J Med 2010;362:648–9.
141. Silbert BS, Scott DA, Evered LA, et al. A comparison of the effect of high- and low-dose fentanyl on the incidence of postoperative cognitive dysfunction after coronary artery bypass surgery in the elderly. Anesthesiology 2006;104: 1137–45.
142. Wang D, Wu X, Li J, et al. The effect of lidocaine on early postoperative cognitive dysfunction after coronary artery bypass surgery. Anesth Analg 2002;95: 1134–41 [Table of contents].
143. Mitchell SJ, Merry AF, Frampton C, et al. Cerebral protection by lidocaine during cardiac operations: a follow-up study. Ann Thorac Surg 2009;87:820–5.
144. Mack WJ, Kellner CP, Sahlein DH, et al. Intraoperative magnesium infusion during carotid endarterectomy: a double-blind placebo-controlled trial. J Neurosurg 2009;110:961–7.
145. Holinski S, Claus B, Alaaraj N, et al. Cerebroprotective effect of piracetam in pa-tients undergoing coronary bypass surgery. Med Sci Monit 2008;14:PI53–7.
146. Slater JP, Guarino T, Stack J, et al. Cerebral oxygen desaturation predicts cogni-tive decline and longer hospital stay after cardiac surgery. Ann Thorac Surg 2009;87:36–44 [discussion: 44–5].
147. Xu T, Bo L, Wang J, et al. Risk factors for early postoperative cognitive dysfunc-tion after non-coronary bypass surgery in Chinese population. J Cardiothorac Surg 2013;8:204.
148. Peng LY, Xu LW, Ouyang W. Role of peripheral inflammatory markers in postop-erative cognitive dysfunction (POCD): a meta-analysis. PLoS One 2013;8: e79624.
149. Van Dijk D, Jansen EW, Hijman R, et al, Octopus Study Group. Cognitive outcome after off-pump and on-pump coronary artery bypass graft surgery: a randomized trial. JAMA 2002;287:1405–12.
150. Kok WF, van Harten AE, Koene BM, et al. A pilot study of cerebral tissue oxygen-ation and postoperative cognitive dysfunction among patients undergoing coronary artery bypass grafting randomised to surgery with or without cardio-pulmonary bypass. Anaesthesia 2014;69:613–22.

151. Siepe M, Pfeiffer T, Gieringer A, et al. Increased systemic perfusion pressure during cardiopulmonary bypass is associated with less early postoperative cognitive dysfunction and delirium. Eur J Cardiothorac Surg 2011;40:200–7.
152. Mathew JP, Mackensen GB, Phillips-Bute B, et al, Neurologic Outcome Research Group of the Duke Heart Center. Effects of extreme hemodilution during cardiac surgery on cognitive function in the elderly. Anesthesiology 2007; 107:577–84.
153. Puskas F, Grocott HP, White WD, et al. Intraoperative hyperglycemia and cognitive decline after CABG. Ann Thorac Surg 2007;84:1467–73.
154. Grigore AM, Grocott HP, Mathew JP, et al, Neurologic Outcome Research Group of the Duke Heart Center. The rewarming rate and increased peak temperature alter neurocognitive outcome after cardiac surgery. Anesth Analg 2002;94:4–10 [Table of contents].
155. Djaiani G, Fedorko L, Borger MA, et al. Continuous-flow cell saver reduces cognitive decline in elderly patients after coronary bypass surgery. Circulation 2007;116:1888–95.
156. Rubens FD, Boodhwani M, Mesana T, et al. The cardiotomy trial: a randomized, double-blind study to assess the effect of processing of shed blood during cardiopulmonary bypass on transfusion and neurocognitive function. Circulation 2007;116:I89–97.
157. Murkin JM, Martzke JS, Buchan AM, et al. A randomized study of the influence of perfusion technique and pH management strategy in 316 patients undergoing coronary artery bypass surgery. II. Neurologic and cognitive outcomes. J Thorac Cardiovasc Surg 1995;110:349–62.
158. Boodhwani M, Rubens FD, Wozny D, et al. Predictors of early neurocognitive deficits in low-risk patients undergoing on-pump coronary artery bypass surgery. Circulation 2006;114:I461–6.
159. Grigore AM, Mathew J, Grocott HP, et al, Neurological Outcome Research Group, CARE Investigators of the Duke Heart Center, Cardiothoracic Anesthesia Research Endeavors. Prospective randomized trial of normothermic versus hypothermic cardiopulmonary bypass on cognitive function after coronary artery bypass graft surgery. Anesthesiology 2001;95:1110–9.
160. Nathan HJ, Wells GA, Munson JL, et al. Neuroprotective effect of mild hypothermia in patients undergoing coronary artery surgery with cardiopulmonary bypass: a randomized trial. Circulation 2001;104:I85–91.
161. Nathan HJ, Rodriguez R, Wozny D, et al. Neuroprotective effect of mild hypothermia in patients undergoing coronary artery surgery with cardiopulmonary bypass: five-year follow-up of a randomized trial. J Thorac Cardiovasc Surg 2007;133:1206–11.
162. Chen MH, Liao Y, Rong PF, et al. Hippocampal volume reduction in elderly patients at risk for postoperative cognitive dysfunction. J Anesth 2013;27:487–92.
163. Messerotti Benvenuti S, Zanatta P, Valfre C, et al. Preliminary evidence for reduced preoperative cerebral blood flow velocity as a risk factor for cognitive decline three months after cardiac surgery: an extension study. Perfusion 2012; 27:486–92.
164. Steinmetz J, Siersma V, Kessing LV, et al, ISPOCD Group. Is postoperative cognitive dysfunction a risk factor for dementia? A cohort follow-up study. Br J Anaesth 2013;110(Suppl 1):i92–7.
165. Zakzanis KK, Mraz R, Graham SJ. An fMRI Study of the Trail Making Test. Neuropsychologia 2005;43(13):1878–86.

Critical Care Issues of the Geriatric Patient

Maurice F. Joyce, MD, EdM, John Adam Reich, MD*

KEYWORDS

- Geriatric critical care • Physiologic effects of aging • End-of-life care • Frailty

KEY POINTS

- Critical care of the geriatric patient is complicated by the interaction of disease with diminished physiologic reserves.
- Frailty, the vulnerable clinical phenotype that makes geriatric patients less able to overcome a stressor, provides a valuable measure of guiding course of care in geriatric patients.
- Improved outcomes in geriatric trauma will depend on geriatric-specific triage, assessment, and treatment protocols.

INTRODUCTION

Caring for critically ill patients in need of life-sustaining support has become a specialty of its own over the last 40 years. Critical care medicine has shown value to patients and care organizations by improving outcomes, controlling cost, and investigating and applying therapy in an evidenced-based manner. Because of changing demographics, critical care of the geriatric patient will become commonplace over the next 30 years. The intensivist must understand physiologic changes associated with aging, manage common comorbid states, and navigate end-of-life care in the geriatric patient. In critical illness, a systems-based approach is used to develop a daily plan, and the same format is used in this article to view the critically ill geriatric patient.

EPIDEMIOLOGY AND IMPACT

In the United States in 2010, there were 40 million people older than 65 years, accounting for roughly 13% of the population.[1] By 2050, an estimated 80 million people, approximately 20% of the population, will be age 65 years or older.[1] A smaller

The authors report no conflicts of interest or disclosures.
Department of Anesthesiology, Tufts Medical Center, 800 Washington Street, Boston, MA 02111, USA
* Corresponding author.
E-mail address: jreich@tuftsmedicalcenter.org

percentage of younger workers are predicted even if current immigration rates remain unchanged, thus placing a greater financial strain on funding the health care system.[1] This inevitable strain has implications for planning intensive care facilities, staffing the workforce, and financing the health care system.

In 2006, approximately 50% of all admissions to intensive care units (ICUs) were elderly patients, and those patients consumed 60% of all ICU days.[2] Further, during the last 6 months of life, ICU days account for 25% of all Medicare dollars spent.[3] This financial burden has caused policy makers to focus on end-of-life spending as a target for bringing health care spending under control. This is a difficult task for the clinician, because it is debatable how much cost savings can really be obtained, because the cost of dying is known only in retrospect.[4] With technological advancement, cost containment will continually be revisited while trying to optimize quality care to the critically ill geriatric population.

NEUROLOGIC SYSTEM

Normal aging results in less brain mass and consequently, less cerebral blood flow.[5] As age increases, cognitive processing time and motor performance slow.[6] The prevalence of dementia increases with age, resulting in half of 85-year-olds having this disease.[6] Although causes of cognitive impairment are varied (including stroke, vascular dementia, and so forth), Alzheimer disease is responsible for 60% to 70%.[7] Cognitive impairment and psychological morbidity can manifest in the ICU as delirium, anxiety, acute stress disorder, and depression.[8] Absence of adaptive devices (hearing aids, eye glasses, dentures) can functionally disable patients and be a contributor to altered mental status in the elderly patient placed in a strange new environment: the ICU.

Pain

Chronic pain is common in the elderly patient, arising from a lifetime of strain from wear-and-tear and common disease states such as osteoarthritis. The prevalence of chronic pain in 85-year-olds reaches 40% to 79%.[9] Despite the high prevalence of chronic pain, acute pain perception in the elderly may be blunted. One study reported less activity in the insular cortex on functional MRI to painful thermal stimulus.[10] This blunted response may be explained by loss of pain and temperature fibers (A-δ) with age.[11] Thus, although acute increases in pain should serve as early warning signs in these patients, pain is less likely to be the presenting symptom in patients with peptic ulcers, myocardial ischemia, postoperative pain, and pneumonia,[12] diagnoses commonly seen in the ICU. Treatment of pain in the ICU is one of the primary functions of the intensivist-led team. Balancing treatment of chronic pain and acute pain from surgery or procedures can be difficult, because of limited physiologic cardiopulmonary reserve. In addition, assessing pain in patients with dementia can be difficult. Patients with dementia may not have cognitive ability to rate pain by number. Further, they have been shown to have increased facial expressions to pain[13] but on the contrary have less change in vital signs when subjected to venopuncture or other noxious stimuli.[14] This author places the postoperative elderly patient on scheduled acetaminophen. This therapy allows for a baseline level of pain control to be achieved without the dangerous side effect profile of opioids. Opioids should be started at 25% to 50% of the recommended adult dose in the elderly.[15] In geriatric patients with minimal fat reserves, fentanyl transdermal patches may be less effective because of impaired absorption. Using nonopioid alternatives such as ketorolac, or weak opioids such as tramadol, is an option for mild to moderate pain, which can also avoid side effects of stronger μ-receptor agonists. Adjunctive medications such as gabapentin can have sedative effects in the elderly, which may be more pronounced during critical illness.

Delirium

Delirium is common in the ICU and when present is associated with longer duration of mechanical ventilation, longer ICU stay, longer hospital stay,[16] and in several studies, increased mortality.[17] Importantly, the causes of delirium are still debated. There are several preexisting factors that predispose patients to delirium: dementia, history of hypertension, history of alcoholism, or a high severity of illness.[18] Physical restraints are most closely associated with delirium,[16] although it is unknown if the presence of restraints is associated with less mobility or behavior that precedes delirium. Pain, agitation, and sedation guidelines by the Society of Critical Care Medicine suggest that benzodiazepine use may predispose patients to delirium.[17] If alternative agents can be used, it is prudent to avoid benzodiazepines in geriatric patients. Treatment with minimal sedation, encouraging sleep–wake cycle, noise reduction, early mobilization, and minimization of restraints have all been used to try to avoid delirium, with mixed results. Antipsychotic therapy has been a main pharmacologic treatment; however, studies show that it has not reduced delirium prevalence or duration.[16] It is better to prevent delirium than to treat it. The most effective means of managing delirium is related to the ICU bundle ABCDE: A for awakening, BC for breathing coordination, D for delirium assessment/management, and E for early exercise/mobility.[19] Early mobility represents a paradigm shift in caring for the critically ill patient. Previously, all medical problems were fixed and patients were hemodynamically normal off vasoactive drugs and tolerating enteral feeds before getting up out of bed. Thinking has now shifted toward early mobility such as walking patients down the hall while they are still dependent on mechanical ventilation. This early mobility can limit muscle wasting and stiffness that is associated with critical illness, in addition to improving mental outlook on recovery. In 1 study,[19] this ABCDE bundle with emphasis on early mobility has resulted in half the amount of delirium as well as 3 days fewer of mechanical ventilation.

Delirium, glucose dysregulation, hypoxemia, sedatives, analgesics, hypotension, and inflammation are all proposed contributors to post-ICU cognitive impairment.[20] It is unclear how to modify all of these factors, but limiting sedation, early mobility, and having a shortened length of stay in the hospital are reasonable goals. A low-cost method for decreasing rate of posttraumatic stress disorder is having staff maintain an ICU diary.[21] This practice allows the patient to go back through the entries and confront or reprocess threatening ICU experiences.[21] Care of the elderly patient also involves caring for their family. A recent study[22] found that the prevalence of depression in informal caregivers of critically ill patients was 75% during an ICU admission, and subsequently 25% a year later.

CARDIOVASCULAR SYSTEM

As individuals age, there is an increasing presence of heart failure, valve disease, and arrhythmias.[23] A decrease in the physiologic reserve of the heart may be unmasked during critical illness, further complicating their management. As the population ages, the incidence of coronary heart disease increases by 26% and mortality by 51%. Cost of coronary care is projected to increase by 41% by 2040.[24]

Arrhythmias

An increase in collagen and fat deposition and a decline in the number of cardiac myocytes occur with age.[25] The conduction system is affected, causing sinus node dysfunction (sick sinus syndrome), atrial fibrillation, and bundle branch blocks. Presence of atrial fibrillation increases with age and reaches 6% by age 80 years.[26] Recently, new onset atrial fibrillation was found to be an independent risk factor for 60-day mortality versus those without atrial fibrillation (51% vs 21%) in the medical ICU.[27] In sepsis, new onset atrial fibrillation is more common in the elderly and was found to be associated with increased length of ICU stay, increased hospital stay, and an increased rate of stroke.[28] New onset atrial fibrillation in the ICU is not just a temporary arrhythmia associated with an underlying disease process but likely is a harbinger of worse outcomes. The presence of sinus node dysfunction, coronary disease, and low ejection fractions leads to implantation of pacemakers and automatic defibrillators. These devices require interrogation during the perioperative period and deactivation in end-of-life situations and can be used to overdrive pace certain arrhythmias or increase heart rate when the intensivist needs more cardiac output.

Valvular Disease

The presence of aortic stenosis increases with age. Symptoms of aortic stenosis can include syncope, dyspnea, and flash pulmonary edema with overhydration. Slow onset of stenosis allows the left ventricle to become hypertrophied, which in conjunction with coronary disease can lead to subendocardial ischemia during exertion. Replacement of the aortic valve is the treatment. Open-heart surgery with cardiopulmonary bypass is considered to be high-risk surgery, which may not be tolerated well in the elderly. However, in 1 case series, elective cardiac surgery was performed safely in patients older than 80 years (3% mortality), but the presence of chronic obstructive pulmonary disease (COPD) or nonelective surgery increased mortality significantly to 14%.[28] Recently, transfemoral percutaneous aortic valve replacements have become a less invasive, viable alternative for aortic valve replacement in elderly patients who are not good candidates for invasive surgery, having an approximately 75% 1-year survival rate.[29] It is important to not only look at survival as the only measure of success, because quality of life scores as well as mortality are now used to grade success of these interventions.[30] At specialized centers, some are now performing these procedures in the catheterization laboratory without general anesthesia, further minimizing cost and length of hospital stay for patients.[30]

Coronary Disease

Aging increases the risk of acute coronary syndrome. Risk factors associated with increased mortality in patients older than 80 years with ST-elevated myocardial infarction include increased cholesterol levels and increased baseline serum creatinine levels.[31] In patients older than 70 years, percutaneous interventions with stents and angioplasty have been shown to be superior to fibrinolytic therapy.[32]

Congestive Heart Failure

Systolic heart failure results from decreased contractility and decreased cardiac output. This condition is managed with afterload reduction (ie, control of hypertension with an angiotensin-converting enzyme inhibitor), low-dose β-blockade if tolerated, and treatment of the underlying cause (ischemic [lifestyle modification, revascularization, statin therapy] versus nonischemic). However, recently, there has been greater focus on heart failure with preserved ejection (formerly known as diastolic heart failure). Heart failure with preserved ejection fraction is highly prevalent in the elderly population, and its prevalence is increasing.[33] Over a lifetime of working, the myocardium becomes stiffer as people age, and although ejection fraction may be preserved, the relaxation of the ventricle can become impaired. People with preserved ejection

fraction and congestive heart failure tended to also have coronary disease, atrial fibrillation, and hypertension compared with those who had systolic heart failure.[33]

Cardiopulmonary Resuscitation

Age does not necessarily have an effect on the neurologic outcome after cardiopulmonary resuscitation (CPR) for cardiac arrests out of hospital.[34] In a French study,[34] time
to performing CPR was most associated with increased survival in the elderly, with
short-term survival being 25%. Long-term cognitive positive outcomes were associated not with age but with the characteristics of CPR (shockable rhythm, lactate level
<5, and lower cumulative dose of epinephrine).[34] Of elderly (>75 years old) survivors of
out-of-hospital CPR and their ICU stay, 75% were alive at 1 year compared with 96%
of the age cohort.[34] CPR should not be limited by age but rather by characteristics of
CPR.

PULMONARY SYSTEM

Respiratory compliance decreases with age as a result of changes in both lung parenchyma and chest wall rigidity.

Respiratory Failure

Geriatric patients with respiratory failure and acute respiratory distress syndrome
recover at the same rate as younger patients but are less likely to be discharged
from the ICU.[35] Pneumococcal pneumonia is primarily a disease of the geriatric patient. A recent analysis showed that in 2040, the demand for hospital admissions as
a result of pneumococcal pneumonia will increase 96% and the annual cost attributed
to this care will be 2.5 billion dollars.[36] In addition to pneumococcal pneumonia, geriatric patients are also admitted to the ICU with congestive heart failure and COPD ex-
acerbations, both of which often require ventilator support. Both of these diagnoses
are shown to have better outcomes when noninvasive mechanical ventilation by
mask rather than endotracheal intubation is used. It is important that this ventilation
be performed in a nonrestrained patient, who can remove the mask if they vomit, or
be performed in an environment with strict monitoring from nurses to avoid
catastrophe.

RENAL SYSTEM

Renal physiology is significantly altered with age. By age 80 years, glomerular filtration
rate is decreased by nearly 45%, as a result of progressive loss of renal tubular mass
and decreased renal blood flow.[37,38] In turn, geriatric patients have a decreased ability
to dilute and concentrate urine in addition to a decreased ability to clear pharmacologic agents. Thus, it is imperative to take this altered physiology into account when
evaluating renal disease in critically ill geriatric patients.

Acute Kidney Injury

Age greater than 65 years has been shown to be an independent risk factor for the
development of acute kidney injury.[39] Importantly, the cause of acute kidney injury
in this population is often multifactorial. It is well known that the incidence of comorbidities significantly increases with age.[40] Notably, cardiovascular disease and
chronic kidney disease greatly increase the risk of acute kidney injury. In addition,
because of these comorbidities, this population is at risk for iatrogenic injury from
pharmacologic exposures and contrast exposure.[41] Thus, the most important factor
in acute kidney injury management is the prevention of this condition. As shown in

Table 1, multiple steps such as hemodynamic optimization and avoidance of nephro-toxic agents can be taken to prevent this injury.[42]

Urinary Tract Infections

Bladder catheters are frequently used in critically ill geriatric patients as a result of immobility and incontinence. Thus, this population is at an increased risk of catheter-associated urinary tract infections and resultant morbidity and mortality.[43] Based on this risk, significant attention has been given to reducing these infections, namely through early discontinuation of catheters and alternative methods such as condom catheters. For example, the use of daily bladder catheter reminders and stop orders has been shown to reduce these infections.[44]

Table 1 Prevention of acute kidney injury in elderly ICU patients	
Hemodynamics	Initiate appropriate monitoring Optimize preload, cardiac systolic or diastolic function, and vascular tone
Volume repletion	Be attentive to signs of hypovolemia Ensure early guided volume repletion Limit use of diuretics and laxatives
Exogenous nephrotoxic	Limit use of all nephrotoxic drugs, in particular nonsteroidal antiinflammatory drugs and aminoglycosides Avoid polypharmacy when possible Avoid combining diuretics with nephrotoxic drugs Adjust dose according to glomerular filtration rate Do not base drug-dosing decisions on absolute creatinine levels Measure drug levels
Contrast medium	Avoid contrast medium, or at least delay contrast use if patient at risk Always use lowest possible quantity of contrast Use hypo-osmolar or iso-osmolar and nonionic contrast Adequate volume repletion (eg, NaCl 0.9%) Bicarbonate infusion possibly beneficial N-acetylcysteine use possibly beneficial
Infection and sepsis	Low index of suspicion for early diagnosis Diagnose/treat sepsis-related intravascular volume depletion, vasoplegia, and cardioplegia Early and appropriate antibiotic initiation Early guided volume repletion, avoid high-molecular-weight hydroxyethyl starch
Perioperative optimization	Differ surgery in at-risk patients if possible Initiate appropriate monitoring (hemodynamic, intra-abdominal pressure) Early and guided optimization of volume status and hemodynamics Limit exposure to nephrotoxins
Abdominal pressure	Measure intra-abdominal pressure in all patients at risk Avoid overresuscitation with fluids Low tidal volume strategy, limit plateau pressure
Mechanical ventilation	Low tidal volume strategy, limit plateau pressure Weaning and extubation as early as possible

From Chronopoulos A, Rosner MH, Cruz DN, et al. Acute kidney injury in elderly intensive care patients: a review. Intensive Care Med 2010;36(9):1459; with permission.

FRAILTY

In the United States, hospital mortality was found to be significantly higher for patients 75 years old and older even after adjusting for organ failure and code status.[23] This finding led the investigators to state that age greater than 75 years should be considered an independent risk factor for death.[23] Besides age, another factor correlated with mortality was preadmission quality of life and functional status.[45] Not surprisingly, there is heterogeneity in the aging population: some have preserved functional status and others are described as frail. Frailty is described as a vulnerable clinical phenotype less able to overcome a stressor.[46] In the elderly, this situation can be caused by loss of physiologic reserve. The frail are significantly less able to return home and are frequently discharged to rehabilitation hospitals. Frail patients have been shown to have worse outcomes in both noncardiogenic surgery and cardiac surgery alike.[46] There are small studies that indicate that the clinical phenotype may be optimized before elective surgery, and larger trials are now under way.[47]

GERIATRIC TRAUMA

Traumatic injuries in the elderly population are associated with significant morbidity and mortality in addition to substantial health care costs and, thus, are a major public health concern. Although physiologic and anatomic alterations in the elderly, as discussed earlier, can account for some of these outcomes, it is clear that improvement is possible. Specifically, geriatric-specific protocols for triage, assessment, and treatment may be helpful.[48]

Triage

In determining the destination for geriatric trauma patients, several factors can play a significant role in outcomes. Matsushima and colleagues[49] reported a correlation between the volume of geriatric patients cared for at a trauma center and lower odds of in-hospital mortality, major complications, and mortality after major complications. In addition, some have advocated for the use of geriatric-specific trauma triage criteria, such as those used in Ohio.[50] Ichwan and colleagues[51] found that these geriatric-specific triage criteria led to a higher sensitivity in identifying those patients who require triage to a level 1 trauma center.

Assessment

Because of baseline physiologic and anatomic alterations in geriatric patients in addition to the frequent presence of multiple comorbidities, it is important to tailor the trauma assessment for these patients. As shown in **Table 2**, the systematic ABCDE method of trauma assessment as taught in advanced trauma life support courses can be modified to more appropriately assess and then subsequently manage these patients.[52] As discussed elsewhere in this review, assessment of frailty can also provide a means for providers to more appropriately predict outcomes in these patients.[53]

Treatment

Because certain traumatic injuries are more common in geriatric patients, there has been increased interest in customizing treatment protocols for these injuries. For example, standardized and methodical approaches to the care of elderly patients with hip fractures have resulted in improved outcomes. These protocols include early mobilization of resources from the emergency department; consideration of hip fractures as surgical emergencies; rapid transfer of these patients to a dedicated geriatric

Table 2
Clinical considerations in the assessment of the geriatric trauma patient

Trauma ABCDE	Clinical Considerations in the Geriatric Trauma Patient
Airway	Macroglossia: upper airway obstruction Lower esophageal sphincter tone: higher risk of aspiration Arthritic process: decreased neck mobility, difficult airway
Breathing	Chest wall rigidity: decreased compliance Costochondral calcification: tendency to rib fractures and its complications Higher closing volume: increases V/Q mismatch
Circulation	Diastolic dysfunction: diastolic heart failure Changes in conduction system: tendency to arrhythmias Poor response to catecholamines: end diastolic volume dependence in stress β-Blocker use: further decrease on catecholamine response Anticoagulants: increase tendency to bleed
Deficit	Thin walls of bridging veins in the dura: prone to tear and lead to subdural hematoma Atherosclerotic plaques in the arterial system: increase likelihood of stroke
Exposure	Skin/thermoregulation changes: hypothermia

Data from Awargal S, Azocar RJ. Trauma and the geriatric patient. In: Barnett SR, editor. Manual of Geriatric Anesthesia. New York: Springer; 2013. p. 193–202.

unit after surgery; and rapid transfer of these patients to a dedicated rehabilitation unit.[54–56]

SUMMARY

"Discharge from the ICU no longer marks the endpoint of critical illness."[57] Postintensive care syndrome refers to the combination of physical and cognitive impairments that persist after the ICU stay that impede the recovery process.[58] In no other age group is that more evident than in the elderly. A patient alive at hospital discharge but transferred to a long-term facility to live in a severely debilitated state for the duration of their life may not be in keeping with the patient's own values. Astoundingly, a review of more than 35,000 Medicare patients showed that those who had been mechanically ventilated during their ICU stay and then discharged from the ICU to a rehabilitation hospital had a 1-year mortality of 57%.[59]

The geriatric patient in the ICU presents a complex interplay between normal loss of physiologic reserve associated with aging, frailty, social factors, and critical illness. It is the job of the intensivist to treat the underlying condition and optimize the patient's physiology to allow for meaningful recovery. Ideally, the primary care physician, family members, and patient would discuss hopes and values before the onset of critical illness; however, this responsibility many times falls on the critical care physician and remains one of their most important and meaningful acts.

REFERENCES

1. Vincent GK, Velkoff VA. The next four decades: The older population in the United States: 2010 to 2050 (No. 1138). US Department of Commerce, Economics and Statistics Administration, US Census Bureau. 2010.
2. Marik PE. Management of the critically ill geriatric patient. Crit Care Med 2006;34: S176–82.

3. Lewis M. Aging demographics and anesthesia. In: Barnett SR, editor. Manual of geriatric anesthesia. 1st edition. New York: Springer; 2013. p. 3–14.

4. Emanuel EJ, Emanuel LL. The economics of dying. The illusion of cost savings at the end of life. N Engl J Med 1994;330(8):540–4.

5. Davis SM, Ackerman RH, Correia JA, et al. Cerebral blood flow and cerebrovascular CO_2 reactivity in stroke age normal controls. Neurology 1983;33(4):391–9.

6. Morris JC, McManus DQ. The neurology of aging: normal versus pathologic change. Geriatrics 1991;46:47–8, 51–4.

7. Cummings JL, Cole G. Alzheimer disease. JAMA 2002;287:2335–8.

8. Karnatovskaia LV. The spectrum of psychocognitive morbidity in the critically ill: a review of the literature and call for improvement. J Crit Care 2015;30(1):130–7.

9. Helme RD, Gibson SJ. The epidemiology of pain in elderly people. Clin Geriatr Med 2001;17(3):417–31.

10. Tseng MT, Chiang MC, Yazhuo K, et al. Effect of aging on the cerebral processing of thermal pain in the human brain. Pain 2013;154:2120–9.

11. Kemp J, Despres O, Pebayle T, et al. Differences in age-related effects on myelinated and unmyelinated peripheral fibres: a sensitivity and evoked potentials study. Eur J Pain 2013;18:482–8.

12. Hadjistavropoulos T, Herr K, Prkachin KM, et al. Pain assessment in elderly adults with dementia. Lancet Neurol 2014;13(12):1216–27.

13. Kunz M, Scharmann S, Hemmeter U, et al. The facial expression of pain in patients with dementia. Pain 2007;133:221–8.

14. Kunz M, Mylius V, Scharmann S, et al. Influence of dementia on multiple components of pain. Eur J Pain 2009;13:317–25.

15. Gupta DK, Avram MJ. Rational opioid dosing in the elderly: dose and dosing intervals when initiating opioid therapy. Clin Pharmacol Ther 2012;91(2):339–43.

16. Mehta S, Cook D, Devlin JW, et al. Prevalence, risk factors, and outcomes of delirium in mechanically ventilated adults. Crit Care Med 2015;43(3):557–66.

17. Ely EW, Shintani A, Truman B, et al. Delirium as a predictor of mortality in mechanically ventilated patients in the intensive care unit. JAMA 2004;291:1753–62.

18. Barr J, Fraser GL, Puntillo K, et al. Clinical practice guidelines for the management of pain, agitation, and delirium in adult patients in the intensive care unit. Crit Care Med 2013;41(1):263–306.

19. Balas MC, Vasilevskis EE, Olsen KM, et al. Effectiveness and safety of the awakening and breathing coordination, delirium monitoring/management, and early exercise/mobility bundle. Crit Care Med 2014;42(5):1024–36.

20. Jackson JC, Mitchell N, Hopkins RO. Cognitive functioning, mental health, and quality of life in ICU survivors: an overview. Psychiatr Clin North Am 2015;38(1):91–104.

21. Mehlhorn J, Freytag A, Schmidt K, et al. Rehabilitation interventions for postintensive care syndrome: a systematic review. Crit Care Med 2014;42(5):1263–71.

22. Haines KJ, Denehy L, Skinner EH, et al. Psychosocial outcomes in informal caregivers of the critically ill: a systematic review. Crit Care Med 2015;43:1112–20.

23. Fuchs L, Chronaki CE, Park S, et al. ICU admission characteristics and mortality rates among elderly and very elderly patients. Intensive Care Med 2012;38(10):1654–61.

24. Odden MC, Coxson PG, Moran A, et al. The impact of the aging population on coronary heart disease in the United States. Am J Med 2011;124(9):827–33.

25. Morley JE, Reese SS. Clinical implications of the aging heart. Am J Med 1989;86:77–86.

26. Furberg CD, Psaty BM, Manolio TA, et al. Prevalence of atrial fibrillation in elderly subjects (the Cardiovascular Health Study). Am J Cardiol 1994;74:236–41.

27. Chen AY, Sokol SS, Kress JP, et al. New-onset atrial fibrillation is an independent predictor of mortality in medical intensive care unit patients. Ann Pharmacother 2015;49:523–7.
28. Gandhi S, Litt D, Narula N. New-onset atrial fibrillation in sepsis is associated with increased morbidity and mortality. Neth Heart J 2015;23(2):82–8.
29. Scandroglio AM, Finco G, Pieri M, et al. Cardiac surgery in 260 octogenarians: a case series. BMC Anesthesiol 2015;15(1):15 eCollection.
30. Agarwal S, Tuzcu EM, Krishnaswamy A, et al. Transcatheter aortic valve replacement: current perspectives and future implications. Heart 2015;101(3):169–77.
31. Claussen PA, Abdelnoor M, Kvakkestad KM, et al. Prevalence of risk factors at presentation and early mortality in patients aged 80 years or older with ST-segment elevation myocardial infarction. Vasc Health Risk Manag 2014;10: 683–9.
32. Assali AR, Moustapha A, Sdringola S, et al. The dilemma of success: percutaneous coronary interventions in patients > or = 75 years of age–successful but associated with higher vascular complications and cardiac mortality. Catheter Cardiovasc Interv 2003;59:195–9.
33. Owan TE, Hodge DO, Herges RM, et al. Trends in prevalence and outcome of heart failure with preserved ejection fraction. N Engl J Med 2006;355(3): 251–9.
34. Grimaldi D, Dumas F, Perier MC, et al. Short and long-term outcome in elderly patients after out-of-hospital cardiac arrest: a cohort study. Crit Care Med 2014; 42(11):2350–7.
35. Ely EW, Wheeler AP, Thompson BT, et al. Recovery rate and prognosis in older persons who develop acute lung injury and the acute respiratory distress syndrome. Ann Intern Med 2002;136:25–36.
36. Wroe PC, Finkelstein JA, Ray GT, et al. Aging population and future burden of pneumococcal pneumonia in the United States. J Infect Dis 2012;205(10): 1589–92.
37. Cook DJ, Rooke GA. Priorities in perioperative geriatrics. Anesth Analg 2003;96: 1823–36.
38. Choudhury DRD, Levi M. Effect of aging on renal function ad disease. Philadelphia: Saunders; 2004.
39. de Mendonca A, Vincent JL, Suter PM, et al. Acute renal failure in the ICU: risk factors and outcome evaluated by the SOFA score. Intensive Care Med 2000; 26:915–21.
40. Pascual J, Liano F, Ortuno J. The elderly patient with acute renal failure. J Am Soc Nephrol 1995;6:144–53.
41. Cheung CM, Ponnusamy A, Anderton JG. Management of acute renal failure in the elderly patient: a clinician's guide. Drugs Aging 2008;25:455–76.
42. Chronopoulos A, Rosner MH, Cruz DN, et al. Acute kidney injury in elderly intensive care patients: a review. Intensive Care Med 2010;36(9):1454–64.
43. Nicolle LE. Catheter-related urinary tract infection: practical management in the elderly. Drugs Aging 2014;31(1):1–10.
44. Meddings J, Rogers MA, Macy M, et al. Systematic review and meta-analysis: reminder systems to reduce catheter-associated urinary tract infections and urinary catheter use in hospitalized patients. Clin Infect Dis 2012;55:923–9.
45. Sacanella E, Pérez-Castejón JM, Nicolás JM, et al. Mortality in healthy elderly patients after ICU admission. Intensive Care Med 2009;35(3):550–5.
46. Bagshaw SM, McDermid RC. The role of frailty in outcomes from critical illness. Curr Opin Crit Care 2013;19(5):496–503.

47. Stammers AN, Kehler DS, Afilalo J, et al. Protocol for the PREHAB study-PRE-operative Rehabilitation for reduction of Hospitalization After coronary Bypass and valvular surgery: a randomised controlled trial. BMJ 2015;5:e007250.
48. Joyce MF, Gupta A, Azocar RJ. Acute trauma and multiple injuries in the elderly population. Curr Opin Anesthesiol 2015;28(2):145–50.
49. Matsushima K, Schaefer EW, Won EJ, et al. Positive and negative volume outcome relationships in the geriatric trauma population. JAMA Surg 2014;149: 319–26.
50. Werman HA, Erskine T, Caterino J, et al. Development of statewide geriatric patients trauma triage criteria. Prehosp Disaster Med 2011;26:170–9.
51. Ichwan B, Darbha S, Shah MN, et al. Geriatric-specific triage criteria are more sensitive than standard adult criteria in identifying need for trauma center care in injured older adults. Ann Emerg Med 2015;65:92–100.
52. Awargal S, Azocar RJ. Trauma and the geriatric patient. In: Barnett SR, editor. Manual of geriatric anesthesia. New York: Springer; 2013. p. 193–220.
53. Joseph B, Pandit V, Sadoun M, et al. Frailty in surgery. J Trauma Acute Care Surg 2014;76:1151–6.
54. Boddaert J, Raux M, Khiami F, et al. Perioperative management of elderly patients with hip fracture. Anesthesiology 2014;121:1336–41.
55. Hip Fracture Accelerated Surgical Treatment and Care Track (HIP ATTACK) Investigators. Accelerated care versus standard care among patients with hip fracture: the HIP ATTACK pilot trial. CMAJ 2014;186:E52–60.
56. Boddaert J, Cohen-Bittan J, Khiami F, et al. Postoperative admission to a dedicated geriatric unit decreases mortality in elderly patients with hip fracture. PLoS One 2014;9:e83795.
57. Needham DM, Feldman DR, Kho ME. The functional costs of ICU survivorship. Collaborating to improve post-ICU disability. Am J Respir Crit Care Med 2011; 183(8):962–4.
58. Denehy L, Elliott D. Strategies for post ICU rehabilitation. Curr Opin Crit Care 2012;18(5):503–8.
59. Wunsch H, Guerra C, Barnato AE, et al. Three-year outcomes for Medicare beneficiaries who survive intensive care. JAMA 2010;303(9):849–56.

Pain Management Issues for the Geriatric Surgical Patient

Jason L. McKeown, MD

KEYWORDS

- Physiology of aging • Opioid risks • Postoperative delirium • Respiratory depression
- Multimodal analgesia • Pain measurement in older adults • Regional anesthesia

KEY POINTS

- The geriatric patient population is the fastest growing segment of society. Members of this group routinely undergo complicated surgical procedures with high levels of postoperative pain that require aggressive treatment.
- Because of complex comorbidities, older patients more commonly have adverse events related to pain therapy and complications related to inadequately treated pain.
- Opioids can be safely used in older adults by reducing dosage and being aware of the unique physiology of the older geriatric patient.
- Certain opioids and nonopioid adjuvants are inappropriate in geriatric patients.
- Careful selection of multimodal agents and use of regional and neuraxial anesthetic techniques can improve postoperative outcomes and reduce opioid-related complications.

The alleviation of pain in the perioperative period has generally been an unattained goal over the last half century since postoperative analgesia began to be studied.[1] However accurate this statement holds across the spectrum of age, it is a proven fact that uncontrolled pain is even more common in older adults, particularly those with cognitive impairment.[2,3] Inadequate analgesia contributes to several adverse postoperative outcomes:

- Cardiopulmonary morbidity
- Longer hospitalization
- Lengthier rehabilitation
- Frequent readmissions
- Development of chronic pain syndromes

The author has no extramural funding or other financial disclosures.
Department of Anesthesiology and Perioperative Medicine, University of Alabama, Birmingham, 619 19th Street South JT862, Birmingham, AL 35249, USA
E-mail address: jmckeown@uab.edu

Anesthesiology Clin 33 (2015) 563–576
http://dx.doi.org/10.1016/j.anclin.2015.05.010   **anesthesiology.theclinics.com**

These factors take on even more serious meaning when applied to the aged patient with multiple comorbidities who is already at increased risk for nosocomial complications (eg, delirium), or who has preexisting functional limitations or problems with chronic pain.[4] For older patients, successful control of pain can significantly alter the postoperative course in a truly positive way.

Uncontrolled pain is the greatest fear of hospitalized patients, be they surgical or nonsurgical.

- The United States geriatric population is growing at an unprecedented rate, with 10,000 individuals reaching the age of 65 every day.
- This population surge mirrors an upward trend over the last decade of increasing numbers of hospitalized geriatric patients.
- In 2007, adults 65 and older comprised only 13% of the United States population but represented 43% of all inpatient hospital days.[5]
- By 2030, the population older than 65 will be 20%.

Common surgical procedures for older adults include elective surgeries such as joint replacements, emergent orthopedic procedures such as fall-related fractures, and surgeries for cancer. All of these are associated with high levels of postoperative pain. As greater numbers of older patients present for complicated surgery over the next decades, anesthesiologists must be prepared to treat pain with ready cognizance of the physiologic changes and comorbidities that are common in the elderly. All those caring for older patients must also be familiar with the safe and appropriate use of analgesic modalities, both pharmacologic and interventional, in the unique context of the older patient.

Given the aging population and increasing number of patients undergoing surgery, all anesthesiologists must be capable of providing expert-level pain treatment for geriatric patients.

RISKS OF PAIN TREATMENT

Older adults are at higher risk for adverse side effects from analgesic treatment in comparison with younger patients, for a variety of reasons.[6] Major areas of risk are listed in **Table 1**. The prevalence of chronic illness and end-organ dysfunction is higher in older adults, but decline in routine organ function is a more specific explanation for increased sensitivity to drugs in the aged. Older adults in the United States take, on average, 5 prescription medications daily; the risk of adverse drug reaction when taking 5 or more is 50%. Pharmacokinetics are altered in a way that predisposes the older adult to drug toxicity. Frail adults are at increased risk not only for side effects and toxicity but also major morbidity and mortality from the complications of analgesics and interventions.

The aged patient with cognitive impairment is at greater risk than cognitively intact patients for undertreatment of pain.[7] Laboratory studies indicate that individuals with cognitive impairment maintain normal pain perception thresholds.[8] Nevertheless, altered central processing of pain stimuli at the cortical level where neurodegenerative deterioration is present alters the way in which pain is expressed by the patient; this is particularly true of the affective component of pain. Because affect and pain behavior strongly influence the clinician's perception of pain, it is easy to understand how significant pain in the cognitively impaired patient could be underappreciated. The type of pain with which a patient presents may also harbor bias toward undertreatment.[9]

Table 1
Major categories of risk for pain therapies in older adults

Risk Category	Mechanism	Example
Decline in organ function	Age-related decline in organ blood flow; slowing of CNS function	Altered metabolism and clearance, especially renally excreted drugs with active metabolites, eg, morphine
Polypharmacy	Higher prevalence of multiple comorbidities	Acute kidney injury, NSAIDs + ACE inhibitors
Pharmacokinetics	Loss of muscle mass; increased adipose. Altered volumes of drug distribution	Lengthened half-life of lipophilic drugs, eg, fentanyl
Drug sensitivity	Decline in cortical mass, decreased drug receptor populations	Delirium related to anticholinergic drugs, eg, meperidine
Frailty	Decline in physiologic reserve to respond to severe complications	Increased mortality from a fall caused by overmedication with opioids

Abbreviations: ACE, angiotensin-converting enzyme; CNS, central nervous system; NSAID, nonsteroidal anti-inflammatory drug.

MEASUREMENT OF PAIN

Appropriate assessment of pain always begins with a complete history and physical examination. Observation of pain behaviors by family members and caretakers provides a useful perspective, but the patient's self-reported pain score provides the most important information. Several well-known pain scoring tools have been validated for use in patients at all stages of cognitive decline (**Table 2**). As cognitive impairment worsens, the assessment of the patient's pain by family and caregivers takes on greater importance.

PHYSIOLOGIC CHANGES IN THE OLDER ADULT

Reduced cardiac output and organ blood flow underlie the pharmacokinetic changes that accompany normal aging. Slowing of the central nervous system (CNS) and alterations in drug metabolism account for most of the sensitivities to analgesics.[10] Impaired excretion of active drug metabolites especially increases the risk of adverse reactions. **Table 3** summarizes these changes, and articles elsewhere in this issue discuss them in more detail.

OPIOID METABOLISM

Opioids are all metabolized in the liver by different processes (**Table 4**). Morphine in older adults has greater potential to cause toxicity because of its active metabolites. Accumulation of these metabolites in patients with renal insufficiency can be harmful, causing respiratory depression, delirium, and myoclonus. In healthy patients receiving typical doses for acute pain, toxicity is unlikely. Opioids with fewer or no active metabolites are preferable in frail patients and those with renal disease.[10] Because elders may have a decline in muscle mass, renal insufficiency may not be reflected by the serum creatinine level. The glomerular filtration rate (GFR) more accurately portrays renal status.

The administration of opioids to older adults with acute pain varies widely in clinical practice, but especially in elders with cognitive dysfunction.[7] Opioid-related

Table 2
Pain scoring tools

Visual Analog Scale	Marks a score on a graded line representing no pain to severe pain	Cognitively intact patients; difficulty speaking
Numeric Rating Scale	0–10 score for no pain to severe pain	Cognitively intact patients; validated in mild to moderate cognitive impairment. Preferred
Verbal Descriptor Scale	Ranks "mild, moderate, severe pain"	Cognitively intact patients; validated in mild to moderate cognitive impairment. Preferred
Faces Scale	Ranks pain on a series of smiling to frowning faces	Validated in mild to moderate cognitive impairment
Pain Assessment Checklist for Seniors with Limited Ability to Communicate Pain Assessment in Advanced Dementia Doloplus-2	—	Validated in severe cognitive impairment
Visual scales, assistive hearing devices	—	Hearing impairment

Data from Falzone E, Hoffmann C, Keita H. Postoperative analgesia in elderly patients. Drugs Aging 2013;30(2):81–90; and Gagliese L, Katz J. Age differences in postoperative pain are scale dependent: a comparison of measures of pain intensity and quality in younger and older surgical patients. Pain 2003;103(1–2):11–20.

Table 3
Physiologic changes in aging

Central nervous system	↓ Cerebral blood flow, ↓ Cortical mass	Altered perception and affective expression of pain
Peripheral nervous system	↓ Blood flow, nerve damage from higher glucose levels	↓ Sensitivity to pain, temperature, touch
Cardiovascular	↓ Cardiac output	↑ Toxicity due to ↑ peak concentration after bolus
Gastrointestinal	↓ Gastric secretions	Impaired dissolution of some drugs. Gut absorption remains normal
Hepatic	↓ Number of hepatocytes, ↓ Cytochrome P450 function, ↓ synthetic function, ↓ serum protein	Impaired metabolism especially demethylation, ↑ drug-drug reactions, ↓ protein binding, ↑ free serum drug level
Renal	↓ Renal blood flow, ↓ GFR	Impaired clearance of metabolites, ↑ half-lives of renally cleared drugs
Musculoskeletal	↓ Muscle mass, ↑ adipose	↓ Water VD, ie, ↑ dose toxicity, hydrophilic drugs; ↑ Fat VD, ie, ↑ half-life lipophilic drugs

Abbreviations: GFR, glomerular filtration rate; VD, volume of distribution.

Table 4 Metabolism of commonly used, preferred opioids in older adults		
Morphine	Conjugation	M3G: neurotoxic M6G: analgesic
Hydromorphone	Conjugation	H3G: neurotoxic, produced in clinically insignificant amounts
Oxycodone	CTP 2D6	Noroxycodone: minimally analgesic Oxymorphone: analgesic, produced in clinically insignificant amounts
Fentanyl	Hydrolysis	No active metabolites
Methadone	N-Demethylation	No active metabolites

complications such as constipation and urinary retention are dose dependent. Delirium has not been shown to be related to dose in some studies.

Neuraxial opioid injections can play an important role in multimodal pain treatment strategies. Advanced age is a risk factor for respiratory depression. When a single intrathecal dose of a hydrophilic opioid such as morphine is injected, very little of the drug is absorbed systemically. Only small amounts may affect rostral brain centers involved in respiration.[11] Like other opioid dosing, a reduction of 25% to 50% is reasonable. Hydromorphone will have less rostral spread than morphine because it is more lipophilic. Spinal analgesia can be extremely effective in abdominal, pelvic, and even chest surgery.

INITIATING TREATMENT

The World Health Organization pain ladder for cancer pain treatment is widely known and is also accepted as a logical treatment approach for postsurgical pain. It is well advised, if possible, to avoid opioids, which carry the highest risk of adverse effect when minor surgery is performed and there is minimal pain. With most major surgery, opioids should be the first line of treatment, and quickly escalated in combination with nonopioid adjuvants for synergistic analgesia and an opioid-sparing effect. "Start low and go slow" is a wise tenet of geriatric medicine. In some cases, however, more aggressive treatment with opioids may decrease the risk for some patients, such as those with dementia in whom uncontrolled pain may drive delirium.[12]

> Start low and go slow—just not too slow! Uncontrolled pain contributes to delirium.

Comorbid depression and other psychological factors can also worsen pain intensity and cause difficulty controlling pain. When initiating therapy, it is very important to continue antidepressants and anxiolytics throughout the perioperative period. Patients may be psychologically, and even physically dependent (carisoprodol) on other adjuvants such as centrally acting muscle relaxants. These drugs have unpredictable effects in older patients and, although they are not recommended by the American Geriatric Society, when a patient is physically dependent it is reasonable to continue but reduce the dose of the drug.

> Continue antidepressants and anxiolytics (and some muscle relaxants) into the perioperative period.

OPIOIDS

Compared with other analgesics, opioids carry the highest side-effect profile. Despite older adults being at greater risk than younger patients for harmful effects of these drugs, opioids are still the mainstay of treatment of severe postoperative pain.

- Opioids are safe for use in the aged.
- Awareness of the physiology and the increased sensitivity of older adults is important.
- Older adults are more sensitive to analgesia, sedation, respiratory depression, cognitive impairment, delirium, and constipation.

Intravenous opioids have the highest risk of adverse events. The intravenous route of administration should be utilized in the immediate postoperative period and the ensuing 24 hours after surgery, or longer if patients must be nil per os. Intravenous patient-controlled analgesia (IVPCA) is the gold standard in successful postoperative analgesia and patient satisfaction. The rationale for IVPCA is to allow patients to achieve their own minimum effective analgesic concentration with smaller but more frequent opioid dosing. Because of the higher risk for adverse events with opioids, this makes IVPCA, with its lower cumulative dose, an attractive technique. IVPCA can even be used safely in carefully selected patients with cognitive impairment.[13]

IVPCA settings and continuous opioid infusions (**Table 5**) are as follows.

- A general rule of thumb is to reduce the starting dose of opioid by half compared with that in a younger patient, and maintain the same dosing interval.[14]
- Continuous intravenous infusions are not advised in unmonitored settings and are not appropriate in opioid-naïve patients.
- Fentanyl's brief duration as a bolus makes it less effective to use without a continuous rate of infusion.
- Lockout settings have not been proved to increase safety and actually may worsen pain outcomes.

The estimated morphine consumption by age in the first 24 hours after major surgery is[15]:

100 − patient's age ≅ mg of intravenous morphine

Because intravenous opioids are associated with a higher risk of adverse events, when the patient is able to resume taking fluids and medications by mouth, oral opioids should be substituted.

- Oral opioids are efficacious for acute pain but slower to act in comparison with the intravenous route.
- All oral opioids take 30 to 60 minutes to reach peak effect.
- All immediate-release opioids for acute pain should be scheduled every 3 to 4 hours.

Table 5
Suggested starting doses for intravenous patient-controlled analgesia

Drug	Dose	Bolus Interval (min)	Loading/Rescue
Morphine	1 mg	10	2 mg every 4 h
Hydromorphone	0.1 mg	10	0.2 mg every 4 h
Fentanyl	10 µg	5	20 µg every 2 h

CHRONIC PAIN AND OPIOIDS IN THE GERIATRIC PATIENT

Chronic pain has a high prevalence in the aged, and the prescription of opioids for all types of chronic pain has risen strikingly over the last decade. Patients who become pharmacologically tolerant to opioids because of chronic therapy have greater difficulty with postoperative pain control. Tolerance to opioids manifests differently from person to person; some older patients may require surprisingly large doses of opioids for effective analgesia.

- The patient who has chronic pain and uses opioid analgesics regularly will require larger doses of analgesics for acute pain control.
- Long-acting opioids for chronic pain should be continued throughout the perioperative period.
- Patients should take their home dose of long-acting opioid on the day of surgery.
- If oral dosing of home medication is not possible, an equianalgesic parenteral substitute should be given.
- Titration of opioids guided by the patient's reported pain intensity should be done while closely monitoring the level of alertness, respiratory rate, and pulse oximetry.

Abruptly stopping a patient's opioid therapy is not recommended because this can lead to delirium, nausea, and vomiting. In particular, tachycardia and hypertension may be dangerous in patients with cardiovascular disease. Reducing chronic opioid dosing is appropriate in cases of:

- Altered mental status
- Opioid-induced toxicity
- Acute decline in renal function
- Respiratory failure

MULTIMODAL ANALGESIA

The role of nonopioids in postsurgical analgesia has been greatly expanded over the past years because of increasing awareness of morbidity attributed to opioids.[16] The effectiveness of opioid analgesia is often offset by adverse effects as described earlier, and the elderly are more sensitive to these. Given their increased analgesic sensitivity to nonopioid adjuvants and opioids alike, the older adult population may benefit than any other group of patients from the synergy of multimodal agents and their opioid-sparing effects more.

NONOPIOID ADJUVANTS
Acetaminophen

Acetaminophen has an excellent history of use in geriatrics. As a nonspecific central cyclooxygenase inhibitor, it has been a useful analgesic for mild to moderate pain for decades. It is very well tolerated in the aged. Acetaminophen has become one of the core components of multimodal analgesic regimens because of its opioid-sparing effect.[17,18]

- No gastrointestinal (GI) disturbance
- Preferred first-line agent for most chronic complaints such as osteoarthritis pain
- Low toxicity risk except in patients with severely impaired liver function
- Hypovolemic surgical patients, malnourished patients, and those with high alcohol consumption are at higher risk for liver damage

- Maximum daily dose in healthy patients 4000 mg
- Reduced dose of 2000 mg in malnourished adults (<50 kg) or with depressed hepatic or renal function

If patients are discharged after surgery on combination analgesics containing acetaminophen, they should be reminded or supervised so as not to exceed the maximum dose of 4000 mg a day. For ease of adherence to a prescribed regimen, it may be best to avoid combination analgesics altogether and instead use a stand-alone drug such as oxycodone. Acetaminophen can then be added as a separate dose, for example, acetaminophen 650 mg every 6 hours. Even if patients exceed the maximum recommended daily dose, it usually takes days to weeks to manifest signs of liver damage.

Nonsteroidal Anti-Inflammatory Drugs

Nonsteroidal anti-inflammatory drugs (NSAIDs) have a well-established role in postoperative pain treatment. In surgeries where peripheral inflammation is a primary pain generator, as in orthopedic surgery, the inhibition of cyclooxygenase enzymes is a potent analgesic mechanism. NSAIDs are effective, but may not be tolerated by both the elderly and their younger counterparts.

- GI disturbances, mucosal bleeding, and ulceration are more common in older adults.
- Use of aspirin, other anticoagulants, or glucocorticoid steroids increases GI risk.
- The cycloxygenase-2 selective drugs (eg, celecoxib) are less associated with GI or bleeding complications.
- All NSAIDs are associated with fluid retention and hypernatremia, which may be dangerous in patients at risk for volume overload, such as those with congestive heart failure (CHF).
- Vasoconstrictive effects increase the risk of ischemia in patients with coronary or cerebrovascular disease.
- In the frail elderly NSAIDs may cause confusion.

Acute kidney injury may occur, and is more likely in anemic or hypovolemic patients. Patients with states of reduced functional blood volume such as occurs in CHF, chronic kidney disease, and diabetes are also at increased risk.[19] The age-related physiologic decline in renal function is best reflected by GFR. Serum creatinine is misleading because of decreased muscle mass. Short-acting NSAIDs are lowest risk. NSAIDs are best avoided in patients with abnormal GFR (<50 mL/min/1.73 m^2) and any of the disease states listed earlier.

Tramadol

Although tramadol is a weak opioid agonist, its lower potency and tricyclic antidepressant properties have led to its inclusion in multimodal plans as a substitute for stronger opioids. It has about one-tenth the potency of morphine and is effective for mild to moderate pain. Similar to codeine, it depends on CYP 2D6 for production of its main active metabolite, O-desmethyl-tramadol.

- Milder analgesic with less respiratory effects
- Possible nausea and delirium in older patients
- Contraindicated in patients with seizures or compromised renal function, which can lead to accumulation
- Because of serotonin/norepinephrine reuptake inhibitory effects, it must be used with caution in patients taking monoamine oxidase inhibitors or other

antidepressants. Complications such as serotonin syndrome are rare, but may occur.

A maximum daily dose of 300 mg is suggested for healthy individuals, with a reduction to 200 mg in patients with other risk factors.[20]

Gabapentinoids

The excellent track record and efficacy of drugs such as gabapentin and pregabalin in chronic neuropathic pain led to their introduction as nonopioid adjuvants in postsurgical pain. Gabapentinoids have been extensively studied and shown to have opioid-sparing effects in a wide variety of surgical procedures including spine surgery, orthopedics, and hysterectomy.[21–23] Analgesic effects are produced by binding to the $\alpha_2\delta$ subunit of neuronal calcium channels.

- Opioid-sparing effect with a single preoperative oral dose
- Must be used with greater caution in the elderly because of dose-dependent sedation
- No metabolism, completely excreted renally
- With physiologic decline in renal function, reduced dosing is appropriate
- Other side effects include dizziness, visual disturbances, cognitive complaints, and swelling of lower extremities

Single preoperative doses of 300 to 400 mg orally are reasonable. The uptake of gabapentin is less predictable than that of pregabalin, which is more potent and bioavailable. Pregabalin also causes less sedation. Gabapentin has been studied as a preventive medication against postoperative delirium, as its opioid-sparing effects were thought to be protective.[24]

WHAT NOT TO USE: THE BEERS CRITERIA

In patients of any age, an adjuvant analgesic should be specifically prescribed based on its efficacy for the type of pain being treated. Certain drugs commonly used for analgesia perioperatively in younger patients present significant risks to older patients. Drugs deemed potentially harmful to elders have been stratified into risk groups by the American Society of Geriatrics in its evidence-based Beers Criteria, which were updated most recently in 2012.[25] The decision to prescribe a particular drug must be individually based on the patient, giving careful consideration to the comorbidities present, the patient's level of tolerance for certain drugs, and the type of pain involved. With these factors in mind the Beers Criteria help guide the clinician in making a full risk-to-benefit assessment for selected agents (**Table 6**).

REGIONAL ANALGESIC TECHNIQUES

With the goals of optimizing analgesia and minimizing systemic adverse effects in older patients, multimodal analgesia is the best practice. Local anesthetics possess the greatest opioid-sparing capacity. In addition to excellent pain relief, regional anesthetic techniques offer other postoperative benefits important to elders: shorter intensive care stays, earlier ambulation, earlier return of bowel function, and improved mental status.[20]

Perineural Blocks

Perineural injections of local anesthetic and the insertion of indwelling catheters for continuous infusion of local anesthetics have become an irreplaceable practice in

Table 6
High-risk medications as per Beers Criteria

Drug	Use	Problem	Recommendation	Alternative
Meperidine	Pain	Anticholinergic effect, delirium, neurotoxic metabolites	Avoid	Other opioid
Antihistamines, eg, diphenhydramine, promethazine	Opioid-related pruritus, nausea	Anticholinergic effect, sedation, delirium	Avoid	Ondansetron, nalbuphine
Muscle relaxants, eg, methocarbamol	Musculoskeletal pain, spasm	Sedation, synergistic with opioids	Avoid	Local therapy, heat, cold, repositioning
Tertiary tricyclic antidepressants, eg, amitriptyline	Neuropathic pain	Anticholinergic effects, sedation, delirium	Avoid	Duloxetine, low-dose gabapentin
Benzodiazepines, eg, diazepam	Anxiety, nausea	Prolonged half-lives, sedation, delirium	Avoid	Low-dose haloperidol

Data from American Geriatrics Society 2012 Beers Criteria Update Expert Panel. American Geriatrics Society updated Beers Criteria for potentially inappropriate medication use in older adults. J Am Geriatr Soc 2012;60(4):616-31.

the treatment of pain after joint replacement and many other types of surgery. New applications are emerging rapidly. With disposable infusion pumps and newer sustained-release liposomal local anesthetics, earlier hospital discharge and more effective physical therapy are possible. Besides portability in ambulatory surgery, perineural blocks offer additional advantages over neuraxial techniques.

- Minimal effect on hemodynamics
- Do not cause urinary retention and there is no need for a bladder catheter, which may be a source of delirium
- Lower risk for hemorrhagic complications with no special considerations for removal of indwelling catheters

Perineural injection techniques are generally low risk in older patients. Local anesthetic toxicity, however, is of special concern:

- Frail elders are at higher risk for local anesthetic toxicity because of lower serum protein levels that cause higher levels of local anesthetic in the plasma.
- End-organ disease, especially cardiac, hepatic, and renal, should be considered, and the lowest volume bolus of anesthetic possible for a particular block should be administered.
- When multiple perineural catheters are used (eg, femoral and sciatic catheters, bilateral transversus abdominis plane block catheters), the total volume of local anesthetic infused should be reduced accordingly.
- Drugs with lower risk for cardiac and CNS toxicity, such as ropivacaine, are most appropriate for continuous infusion.

Perineural injections may be more technically challenging in some older patients:

- Patients with acute trauma such as hip fractures may be difficult to position for blocks, and the risk-to-benefit ratio of sedation, especially with benzodiazepines, must be considered. Small doses of fentanyl and propofol are useful.
- Loss of muscle mass and poor tissue echogenicity may cause poor visualization of nerves with ultrasonography.
- Obesity in older adults makes challenging the identification of nerves with surface landmarks and nerve stimulator techniques.
- Bedbound patients need vigilant surveillance of indwelling catheter sites for potential skin breakdown.

Some special considerations should be given to older adults with cognitive impairment who are discharged home with blocks and indwelling catheters. Caregiver support at home should be capable of handling several potential problems:

- Supervision of indwelling catheter so that patient does not pull it out prematurely
- Problems such as leakage at the catheter site must be dealt with to avoid causing agitation or confusion
- Motor blockade from lower extremity blocks can lead to falls

When regional blockade recedes after a single dose of anesthetic, or a catheter is removed, an oral analgesic plan appropriate for the patient's age and comorbidities must be ready. Education of the patient and family must also give specific instructions if a catheter migrates outward unexpectedly. Steps should include oral analgesics and emergency contact numbers if analgesics fail to control the pain.

Neuraxial Techniques

Epidural analgesia has a 3-decade history of proven superior pain relief and improved outcomes compared with conventional methods of systemic opioid delivery. The epidural route of administration for opioid, local anesthetic, or a combination provides superior analgesia for dynamic or rest pain in comparison with systemic opioids.[26] Elderly patients having a higher burden of comorbidities and requiring more complicated surgeries stand to benefit more than younger patients from epidural analgesia. Unfortunately, technical difficulties, the use of anticoagulant drugs in the perioperative period, and the logistical requirements for postoperative management of catheters often prevent older patients from receiving epidural analgesia.

Although improved outcomes shown in studies have not been exclusively demonstrated in older patients, several end points are beneficial to older patients[27,28]:

- Earlier ambulation
- Earlier return of bowel function
- Earlier return of mental capacity
- Shorter hospitalization
- Lowered cardiovascular morbidity

Most of the benefits are due to opioid-sparing effects of local anesthetic and the abolition of the surgical stress response, which leads to many harmful downstream effects. Effects on bowel motility are limited to epidurals that are placed at the thoracic level. Local anesthetic drugs alone alter the stress response; epidural opioids do not.[29]

Combination of low-dose opioid and local anesthetic is most appropriate for limiting the toxic effects of each drug. Just as older adults are more sensitive to systemic opioids, they have increased sensitivity to spinal opioids. Surprisingly, low-dose opioids administered epidurally produce profound analgesia. Elderly patients are also more sensitive to the effects of local anesthetics within the epidural space. Smaller infusion volumes spread much more widely in older individuals. The risk of extended cephalocaudal spread is a more pronounced sympathectomy and, subsequently, hypotension. Bolus doses must be reduced to compensate for this. Careful catheter placement at the spinal level that corresponds to the surgical dermatome will help limit the volume required for coverage of the incision.

SUMMARY

The treatment of postoperative pain of the older adult patient is critically important to a good outcome after surgery. Because of aging physiology, complex comorbidities, high prevalence of chronic pain, and the nature of surgical procedures, the task of pain management is sometimes difficult in older patients. A multimodal analgesic approach with nonopioids and regional techniques is essential to help limit opioid-related complications such as respiratory depression and delirium. Consideration of side effects of medications and complications related to interventional techniques must be thorough. Starting with lower doses and titrating conservatively are important. Extra vigilance and proactive planning are required to avoid complications related to problems of polypharmacy, cognitive decline, and frailty.

REFERENCES

1. Gan TJ, Habib AS, Miller TE, et al. Incidence, patient satisfaction, and perceptions of post-surgical pain: results from a US national survey. Curr Med Res Opin 2014;30(1):149–60.

2. The management of chronic pain in older persons: AGS panel on chronic pain in older persons. American Geriatrics Society. J Am Geriatr Soc 1998;46(5):635–51.
3. Schofield PA. The assessment and management of peri-operative pain in older adults. Anaesthesia 2014;69(Suppl 1):54–60.
4. Falzone E, Hoffmann C, Keita H. Postoperative analgesia in elderly patients. Drugs Aging 2013;30(2):81–90.
5. Hall MJ, DeFrances CJ, Williams SN, et al. National Hospital Discharge Survey: 2007 summary. Natl Health Stat Report 2010;(29):1–20, 24.
6. Popp B, Portenoy R. Management of chronic pain in the elderly: pharmacology of opioids and other analgesic drugs. In: IASP, Task Force on Pain in the Elderly, Ferrell B, Ferrell BA, editors. Pain in the elderly : a report of the Task Force on Pain in the Elderly of the International Association for the Study of Pain. Seattle (WA): IASP Press; 1996. p. 21–34.
7. Mehta SS, Siegler EL, Henderson CR Jr, et al. Acute pain management in hospitalized patients with cognitive impairment: a study of provider practices and treatment outcomes. Pain Med 2010;11(10):1516–24.
8. Scherder E, Oosterman J, Swaab D, et al. Recent developments in pain in dementia. BMJ 2005;330(7489):461–4.
9. Hwang U, Belland LK, Handel DA, et al. Is all pain is treated equally? A multicenter evaluation of acute pain care by age. Pain 2014;155(12):2568–74.
10. Baillie SP, Bateman DN, Coates PE, et al. Age and the pharmacokinetics of morphine. Age Ageing 1989;18(4):258–62.
11. Slappendel R, Weber EW, Dirksen R, et al. Optimization of the dose of intrathecal morphine in total hip surgery: a dose-finding study. Anesth Analg 1999;88(4):822–6.
12. Morrison RS, Magaziner J, Gilbert M, et al. Relationship between pain and opioid analgesics on the development of delirium following hip fracture. J Gerontol A Biol Sci Med Sci 2003;58(1):76–81.
13. Licht E, Siegler EL, Reid MC. Can the cognitively impaired safely use patient-controlled analgesia? J Opioid Manag 2009;5(5):307–12.
14. Pasero CL, McCaffery M. Managing postoperative pain in the elderly. Am J Nurs 1996;96(10):38–45 [quiz: 46].
15. Macintyre PE, Schug SA. Acute pain management: a practical guide. Edinburgh (United Kingdom); New York: Elsevier Saunders; 2007.
16. Buvanendran A, Kroin JS. Multimodal analgesia for controlling acute postoperative pain. Curr Opin Anaesthesiol 2009;22(5):588–93.
17. Toms L, McQuay HJ, Derry S, et al. Single dose oral paracetamol (acetaminophen) for postoperative pain in adults. Cochrane Database Syst Rev 2008;(4):CD004602.
18. Moon YE, Lee YK, Lee J, et al. The effects of preoperative intravenous acetaminophen in patients undergoing abdominal hysterectomy. Arch Gynecol Obstet 2011;284(6):1455–60.
19. Mamdani M, Juurlink DN, Lee DS, et al. Cyclo-oxygenase-2 inhibitors versus non-selective non-steroidal anti-inflammatory drugs and congestive heart failure outcomes in elderly patients: a population-based cohort study. Lancet 2004;363(9423):1751–6.
20. Pasero C, Rakel B, McCaffery M. Postoperative pain management in the older adult. In: Gibson SJ, Weiner DK, editors. Pain in older persons, vol. 35. Seattle (WA): IASP Press; 2005. p. 377–95.
21. Chang CY, Challa CK, Shah J, et al. Gabapentin in acute postoperative pain management. Biomed Res Int 2014;2014:631756.

22. Kong VK, Irwin MG. Gabapentin: a multimodal perioperative drug? Br J Anaesth 2007;99(6):775–86.
23. Seib RK, Paul JE. Preoperative gabapentin for postoperative analgesia: a meta-analysis. Can J Anaesth 2006;53(5):461–9.
24. Leung JM, Sands LP, Rico M, et al. Pilot clinical trial of gabapentin to decrease postoperative delirium in older patients. Neurology 2006;67(7):1251–3.
25. American Geriatrics Society 2012 Beers Criteria Update Expert Panel. American Geriatrics Society updated Beers Criteria for potentially inappropriate medication use in older adults. J Am Geriatr Soc 2012;60(4):616–31.
26. Block BM, Liu SS, Rowlingson AJ, et al. Efficacy of postoperative epidural analgesia: a meta-analysis. JAMA 2003;290(18):2455–63.
27. Park WY, Thompson JS, Lee KK. Effect of epidural anesthesia and analgesia on perioperative outcome: a randomized, controlled Veterans Affairs cooperative study. Ann Surg 2001;234(4):560–9 [discussion: 569–71].
28. Moraca RJ, Sheldon DG, Thirlby RC. The role of epidural anesthesia and analgesia in surgical practice. Ann Surg 2003;238(5):663–73.
29. Kehlet H, Holte K. Effect of postoperative analgesia on surgical outcome. Br J Anaesth 2001;87(1):62–72.

Chronic Pain in Older Adults

Mark C. Bicket, MD*, Jianren Mao, MD, PhD

KEYWORDS

- Chronic pain • Persistent pain • Older adults • Geriatrics • Pain management
- Pain clinics • Aging • Aged

KEY POINTS

- Chronic pain ranks among one of the most common, costly, and incapacitating conditions in later life.
- Chronic pain does not constitute part of the normal aging process, contrary to beliefs among the public and physicians that pain is an unavoidable consequence of getting older.
- Increasing age causes physiologic abnormalities including an increase in pain threshold, a decrease in pain tolerance, and alterations in pharmacokinetics and pharmacodynamics that increase the risk of side effects from pharmacologic treatment.
- Unique features to pain assessment in older adults include the likelihood of multiple diagnoses contributing to chronic pain, the ability to use self-report in older adults including most who have mild to moderate cognitive impairment, and the recognition that older adults with cognitive impairment may demonstrate a variety of behaviors to communicate pain.
- The management of chronic pain in older adults is best accomplished through a multi-modal approach, including pharmacologic and nonpharmacologic treatments, physical rehabilitation, and psychological therapies. Interventional pain therapies may be appropriate in select older adults and may reduce the need for pharmacologic treatments.

INTRODUCTION

Chronic pain ranks among one of the most common, costly, and incapacitating conditions in later life.[1] Although the prevalence of acute pain remains similar across the adult years of life, the prevalence of chronic pain increases in an age-related manner

Disclosure: The authors have no financial conflicts of interest to disclose.
Department of Anesthesia, Critical Care, and Pain Medicine, Massachusetts General Hospital, Harvard Medical School, Wang Ambulatory Care Center, 55 Fruit Street Gray-Bigelow 444, Boston, MA 02114, USA
* Corresponding author. Wang Ambulatory Care Center, Suite 340, 15 Parkman Street, Boston, MA 02114.
E-mail address: mbicket@partners.org

up to at least the seventh decade[2,3] but seems to plateau among age groups older than 65 when adjusting for other comorbidities and characteristics.[4]

Painful conditions are one of the most common reasons that older persons seek health care in the ambulatory setting (**Box 1**).[5] Arthritis-related diagnoses stand atop the list of painful conditions affecting older adults, as more older adults report low back pain in comparison with adults 18 years of age or older (**Fig. 1**). Prescription medication use for pain is higher among adults 65 years of age or older than in younger persons, and the percentage of older adults on at least 1 prescription medication for pain increased at a faster rate over the past 2 decades in comparison with other age groups (**Fig. 2**). Bothersome pains in older persons disproportionately affect women more than men, and more than 50% of community-dwelling older persons report such pain on a regular basis.[4] In the residential care setting, more than 80% of nursing home residents report chronic pain.[6]

Chronic pain does not constitute part of the normal aging process, contrary to beliefs among the public and physicians that pain is an unavoidable consequence of getting older.[7,8] Despite its high prevalence, pain among older persons is almost always the result of pathology involving a physical or psychological process. Combating the myth and misunderstanding that "pain is inevitable with aging" represents one of the educational challenges to permit a cultural transformation of the approach to pain treatment in older persons.[1,9]

AGE-RELATED DIFFERENCES RELEVANT TO PAIN

Changes in pain perception among older adults result from an aging process that affects functioning at the cellular, tissue, organ, system, and population levels. Some underlying processes seem similar across all older adults, but aging is not a uniform process. Older persons demonstrate significant variation among individual responses to aging.[10] The heterogeneity that exists among the physiologic,

---

Box 1
Common causes of chronic pain in older persons

Arthritis and related arthritides

  Osteoarthritis

  Rheumatoid arthritis

Spinal canal stenosis

Diabetic peripheral neuropathy

Trigeminal neuralgia

Postherpetic neuralgia (shingles)

Cancer-related pain

  Chemotherapy-induced peripheral neuropathy

  Radiation-induced neuropathy

Peripheral vascular disease

Central poststroke pain

Myofascial pain

Fibromyalgia

Postsurgical pain

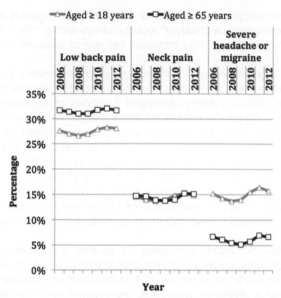

Fig. 1. Adults with pain during the past 3 months. Percentage based on 3-year moving average for low back pain, neck pain, and severe headache or migraine by year from 2006 to 2012. Percentage endorsing pain for individuals aged 18 years and older and 65 years and older is represented by triangles and squares, respectively. Estimates for 18 years and older are age adjusted. (*Data from* Health, United States. Centers for Disease Control and Prevention. 2013. Available at: http://www.cdc.gov/nchs/hus/contents2013.htm; and the National Health Interview Survey, 2015. Accessed February 28, 2015.)

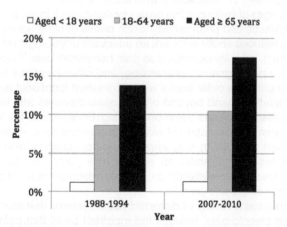

Fig. 2. Prescription drug use for pain in the past 30 days. Percentage of population reporting use of 1 or more prescription medications for pain in the past 30 days by age group. Percentages for younger than 18 years, 18 to 64 years, and aged 65 years and older are represented by white, gray, and black bars, respectively. The increase in prescription drug use for pain between the 2 periods increased at a higher rate for persons aged 65 and older (27%) compared with persons aged 18 to 64 (22%) or younger than 18 years (8%). (*Data from* Health, United States. Centers for Disease Control and Prevention. Analgesic prescriptions. 2013. Available at: http://www.cdc.gov/nchs/hus/contents2013.htm; and National Health and Nutrition Examination Survey, 2015. Accessed February 28, 2015.)

psychological, and functional capacities of older persons suggests what is clinically apparent when comparing a "healthy" octogenarian with a "frail" septuagenarian: chronologic advances in age may increase the risk of disease, but aging itself is not a disease.[11]

Pain signal changes associated with aging include decreases in both molecular and cellular elements that participate in the normal function of nociceptive pathways. In the peripheral nervous system, damaged functions of nociceptive nerves may result from a loss of integrity or decreased density of cellular elements, as suggested by decreases in concentrations of Substance P and calcitonin gene-related peptide.[12] In the central nervous system, reductions in several critical lines of neurotransmission (including endorphins, γ-aminobutyric acid, serotonin, norepinephrine, opioids, and acetylcholine, among others) likely result in inadequate neurochemicals to facilitate proper pain signal transmission and neuromodulation.[13] Evidence also suggests that aging results in dysfunction of the descending modulatory pathways of the spinal dorsal column, which normally serve as an endogenous pain inhibitory system.

Alterations in pain perception with aging are an area of contention among several studies, but a large meta-analysis suggests that among older adults the pain threshold increases and pain tolerance decreases.[14] The threshold for pain may vary based on the type of stimulus (increase with heat, no change with electrical stimulation, decrease with mechanical pressure and ischemia), duration (increase with shorter duration), and location (increase at peripheral or visceral site).[13,15,16] Although pain may not serve as a reliable warning sign of tissue damage in some atypical clinical presentations (cardiac ischemic pain, abdominal pain) because of the increased pain threshold, this finding should not lead to the conclusion that most of the older adult population will not experience pain.[17,18] Rather, the increased pain threshold that accompanies aging may imply that more significant levels of underlying pathologic disorder may be present in older adults who endorse pain.

Physiologic changes of various aging organ systems result in implications important for the pharmacokinetic and pharmacodynamic profile of older adults (**Table 1**). With age also comes a reduced ability to mount an adequate physiologic response to stress associated with pain, a quality described as pain homeostenosis.[13] Consequently, the effects of aging on pain signaling, processing, and other functions relevant to analgesia are more apparent in older adults with diminished functional reserve. Stresses placed on older adults expand beyond organ-based diseases and into relationship- and population-based transitions common to aging. For example, the loss of a spouse or a close family member, cessation of work through retirement or termination, or the loss of independent functioning may impair an older person's ability to cope with ongoing pain or reduce the ability to endure new pain. Chronic pain may also contribute to impaired family relationships, directly affecting the adult children of older adults who experience chronic pain.[19]

Aging also introduces a variety of distorted belief systems that must be addressed effectively to treat chronic pain. Besides the incorrect belief that pain is an unavoidable consequence of getting older, additional misconceptions include the assumption that treatment of chronic pain will be unlikely to provide any benefit.[9] Older adults may also have difficulty providing accurate recall of pain in the past days or weeks, may misinterpret symptoms resulting from pain as a result of another process (such as depression), and may engage in stoicism by being unwilling to disclose their pain to others.[20] These challenges highlight the need for an assessment of chronic pain in the older adult population that differs from that of younger people.

Table 1
Physiologic changes related to pharmacokinetics and pharmacodynamics in older adults

Characteristic	Age-Related Change	Impact
Pharmacokinetics		
Absorption	↑ Gastric pH ↓ Secretory capacity ↓ Gastrointestinal blood flow	Minimal clinical impact in rate or amount of drug absorption, with exception of rectal route (variable change)
Distribution	↑ Body fat	↑ V_D for lipophilic drugs, requiring often undesirable ↑ dosing
	↓ Total body water	↓ V_D for hydrophilic drugs, so ↓ dosing needed
	↓ Plasma albumin ↓ Protein affinity	↓ V_D for highly protein bound drugs, so ↓ dosing needed
Metabolism	↓ liver blood flow, mass, and volume	—
	↓/↔ First-pass metabolism ↓ Phase I metabolism (oxidation)	↑ Bioavailability of drugs with first-pass and phase I metabolism
	↔ Phase II metabolism (conjugation)	Metabolism of most opioid medications (via conjugation) is preserved
Elimination	↓ Glomerular filtration rate ↓ Renal blood flow	↓ clearance and ↑ $t_{1/2}$ of drugs with renal elimination
Pharmacodynamics		
Central nervous system	↓ Brain blood flow, mass, and volume	—
Peripheral nervous system	↓ Density of myelinated and unmyelinated fibers ↑ No. of damaged nerve fibers	Unclear impact on pain threshold and tolerance
Receptors	↓ Receptor density ↑ Receptor affinity	↓ dosing needed and ↑ risk of side effects

↑, increased; ↓, decreased; ↔, unchanged; $t_{1/2}$, half-life; V_D, volume of distribution.
Adapted from Mitchell SJ, Hilmer SN, McLachlan AJ. Clinical pharmacology of analgesics in old age and frailty. Rev Clin Gerontol 2009;19:106; with permission.

PAIN ASSESSMENT IN OLDER ADULTS

Effective treatment of chronic pain requires a meaningful assessment of pain in the older adult. A comprehensive history and physical examination, along with consideration for the use of diagnostic procedures, will permit interventions of disease-modifying conditions to alleviate identifiable source(s) of pain.[21] Diagnostic imaging and ancillary tests should only be obtained based on clinical and physical examination findings, given the increasing incidence of incidental findings in asymptomatic older adults.[22] In cases where no definable disorder concordant with chronic pain is apparent, pain should be recognized as a legitimate but discrete clinical entity, and treated accordingly.[23]

Older adults likely have more than one diagnosis that contributes to chronic pain, and because this population does not adhere to the law of parsimony (Occam's razor), addressing multiple sources of pain through comprehensive evaluations is necessary to alleviate pain.[24] In addition, the diminished physiologic reserve and loss of pain as a warning sign in some older adults may increase the likelihood of atypical presentations of chronic pain.[25]

The best indicator of pain in older adults remains a person's self-reported pain level, and several assessment tools for pain intensity are both useful and valid in this population (**Table 2**).[26] Mild to moderate cognitive impairment, common to conditions such as dementia, does not impair the appropriate use of these tools in most situations.[27] Older adults with cognitive impairment may demonstrate a variety of behaviors to communicate pain, including facial expressions, verbalization, body movements, and changes in interactions with other people and their environment (**Box 2**). Given the variation in pain behaviors with cognitive impairment, pain may be underappreciated and undertreated in this population.[25] Assessing pain levels or behaviors is most effectively performed during a movement-based task or when compared with a preexisting baseline state.[26] In addition, caregivers may provide ancillary information relevant to pain assessment for adults with cognitive impairment.

Outcomes measures besides pain level provide important information regarding the impact of chronic pain and its treatment in all populations, but especially in older adults. Assessment of functional status including activities of daily living, mobility, sleep, appetite, weight changes, mood (including screening for anxiety, depression, and risk of suicide), and cognitive impairment (dementia or delirium) is necessary.[26] Adequate pain management is expected to result in improvements in 1 or more of these domains, as untreated or undertreated pain may contributes to or worsens the conditions in these domains.[28]

PAIN MANAGEMENT IN OLDER ADULTS

The management of chronic pain in the older adult is best accomplished through a multimodal approach that builds on stepwise interventions, including pharmacologic and nonpharmacologic treatments, physical rehabilitation, and a strong patient-physician relationship (**Box 3**).[29] To adequately address chronic pain, adults in later life benefit from involvement of a multidisciplinary team including the geriatrician and pain medicine specialist, in addition to a pain psychologist or psychiatrist, physical and occupational therapist, and rheumatologist when appropriate. Collaborative care interventions for chronic pain in older adults have been shown to improve a variety of outcome measures, including reductions in pain-related disability, pain intensity, and depression, in comparison with usual treatment.[30] However, some evidence suggests that older adults have historically experienced an age-related bias limiting referral for pain treatment,[31] and older adults demonstrate more physical problems than younger adults on initial presentation to pain management programs.[32] Available resources for clinicians include treatment guidelines and reviews focusing on older adults, which provide useful frameworks to guide pain management in later life.[6,26,28,29,33,34]

Pharmacologic approaches represent one treatment modality that should complement nonpharmacologic approaches to help achieve specific patient goals such as improved quality of life or greater functional status (**Box 4**).[28] Avoiding the use of inappropriate and high-risk drugs in older adults serves as a safeguard to minimize the likelihood of adverse drug events and other medication-related problems (**Table 3**).[33] Older adults are not immune from harmful modern trends in pharmacologic management, as evidenced by the opioid overdose epidemic with a 4-fold increase in opioid drug-poisoning deaths in those aged 65 years and older in the 10-year period leading up to 2010 (**Fig. 3**). The higher risk of side effects of pain medications with increasing age highlights the appeal of nonpharmacologic approaches.

Interventional pain therapies such as image-guided nerve blocks, nerve ablation, and other minimally invasive procedures constitute another possible treatment

Table 2
Assessment scales for older persons with persistent pain

Instrument	Description	Item(s)	Abstract Thinking	Comments
Numeric rating scale (NRS)	Numerical rating via an 11-point scale, ranging from 0 (no pain) to 10 (worst pain)	Numbers: ranging from 0 (no pain) to 10 (worst pain)	Moderate	Appropriate first-line pain-rating instrument in cognitively intact older persons Moderate abstract thinking
Visual analog scale (VAS)	Continuous rating via designating a position along a line	Position designated along line between 2 end points (no pain, worst possible pain)	Significant	Ideal for research given wide range of applicable statistical methods Use of pencil/paper or device to designate position is cumbersome for frail older persons Significant abstract thinking
Verbal rating scale (VRS) or verbal descriptor scale (VDS)	Verbal rating via 4-item categorical scale Instruments up to 7 items available	Descriptions: "none," "mild," "moderate," "severe"	Moderate	Limited number of responses and higher language demand Easy to use in clinical environment but insufficient for research purposes Moderate abstract thinking
Facial pain scale (FPS)	Pictorial rating via 6-item categorical scale 7-, 9-, and 11-item instruments available	Drawings: a series of faces arranged in order of increasing pain expressions	Moderate	Validated in older persons including minority groups Moderate abstract thinking
Pain thermometer	Verbal rating via 6-item categorical scale arranged in vertical order adjacent to image of a thermometer	Descriptions: ranging from "no pain"/white color at base to "pain as bad as could be"/red color at top	Minimal	Validated in older persons with cognitive impairment Minimal abstract thinking

---

Box 2
Common pain behaviors in cognitively impaired older persons

Facial Expressions

Frown; sad, frightened face

Grimace, wrinkled forehead, closed or tightened eyes

Rapid blinking

Verbalizations, Vocalizations

Sighing, moaning, groaning, grunting

Calling out, asking for help

Noisy breathing, verbally abusive

Body Movements

Rigid, tense body posture, guarding

Fidgeting, increased pacing, rocking

Restricted movement, gait or mobility changes

Changes in Interpersonal Interactions

Aggressive, combative, resisting care

Decreased social interactions

Socially inappropriate, disruptive, withdrawn

Changes in Activity Patterns or Routines

Refusing food, appetite change

Sleep, rest pattern changes

Sudden cessation of common routines

Increased wandering

Mental Status Changes

Crying or tears

Increased confusion

Irritability or distress

From AGS Panel on Persistent Pain in Older Persons. Management of persistent pain in older persons. J Am Geriatr Soc 2002;50:S211; with permission.

---

modality in older adults with chronic pain.[6] Older adults with cancer who demonstrate increasing opioid requirements may benefit from administration of opioid via an intrathecal drug delivery system.[35] Analgesia provided by interventional therapies may lead to a reduction in pain medication use and side effects in appropriately selected older adults. The presence of persistent pains, including low back pain in the sacroiliac joint or lumbar facet column, radicular pain in any extremity, or hip pain, warrants further evaluation for consideration of interventional therapy.[36] Given the increasing probability of comorbidities and anticoagulation in older adults, special attention must be devoted to the risk/benefit profile of these procedures in comparison with that of discontinuation of antiplatelet or anticoagulation medication (ie, possible thrombosis).[37] Interventions may provide pain relief that permits an older adult to more fully engage in rehabilitation and other activities that increase their quality of life.

Box 3

Key points regarding overall approach to management of persistent pain in the older adult

1. Determine patient's comorbidities, cognitive and functional status, treatment goals and expectations, and social and family supports before initiating treatment

2. Intervene using a multimodal approach, including pharmacologic and nonpharmacologic treatments in addition to physical and occupational rehabilitation modalities

3. Develop and enrich therapeutic alliance between patient and physician (physician must respond promptly and reliably to patient calls and provide backup coverage when away; consider all patient input seriously; encourage hope without overpromising therapeutic success)

4. Be willing to revisit previously used pharmacologic and nonpharmacologic treatment modalities with indicated modifications

5. Involve and engage caregivers and seek out other resources (eg, community-based programs) that can help to reinforce treatment adherence and maintain treatment gains

6. Reinforce positive outcomes at each visit

From Makris UE, Abrams RC, Gurland B, et al. Management of persistent pain in the older patient: a clinical review. JAMA 2014;312:827; with permission.

Box 4

Key points regarding pharmacologic and nonpharmacologic approaches

1. Link potential treatment benefits with important patient goals (eg, increased ability to perform activities of daily living)

2. Use medication combinations (in which each analgesic works by a different mechanism) to enhance analgesic effectiveness

3. Acetaminophen remains first-line pharmacologic treatment for older adults with mild to moderate pain

4. Avoid long-term use of oral nonsteroidal anti-inflammatory drugs, given their significant cardiovascular, gastrointestinal, and renal risks

5. Trial of opioid is appropriate for patients not responsive to first-line therapies and who continue to experience significant functional impairment due to pain

6. Consider serotonin-norepinephrine reuptake inhibitors or selective serotonin reuptake inhibitors in patients with comorbid depression and pain

7. Implement surveillance plan (ie, efficacy, tolerability, adherence) with each new treatment

8. Physical activity (including physical therapy, exercise, or other movement-based programs such as tai chi) constitutes a core component of managing persistent pain in older patients

9. Educate older patients about safety and efficacy of cognitive-behavioral and movement-based therapies and identify local practitioners or agencies that provide them

10. Determine whether treatment goals are being met; if goals are not met, medication should be tapered and discontinued, physical and occupational therapy prescription modified, or both

From Makris UE, Abrams RC, Gurland B, et al. Management of persistent pain in the older patient: a clinical review. JAMA 2014;312:827; with permission.

Table 3
Beers list: potentially inappropriate pain and pain-related medication use in older adults

Drug	Adverse Effects
NSAIDs	
Indomethacin (Indocin, Incodin SR)	Of all NSAIDs, most significant central nervous system (CNS) side effects
Ketorolac (Toradol), including parenteral	Gastrointestinal bleeding and peptic ulcer disease
Oral non-COX–selective NSAIDs Aspirin >325 mg/d Diclofenac (Voltaren, Flector) Etodolac (Lodine) Ibuprofen (Advil, Motrin) Meloxicam (Mobic) Nabumetone (Relafen) Naproxen (Naprosyn, Aleve)	Long-term use of non-COX–selective NSAIDs increases risk of GI bleeding and peptic ulcer disease Particular caution with age >75 or concomitant use of corticosteroids, anticoagulants, or antiplatelet agents Risk of renal failure, hypertension, and congestive heart failure
Opioids	
Meperidine (Demerol)	Ineffective oral analgesic at commonly used dosages Renally cleared metabolite may cause seizures and death
Pentazocine (Talwin)	Opioid analgesic that causes adverse CNS effects, including confusion and hallucinations, more commonly than other narcotic drugs
Tricyclic Antidepressants	
Amitriptyline (Elavil) Doxepin at >6 mg/d (Silenor, Zonalon, Prudoxin) Chlordiazepoxide-amitriptyline (Limbitrol) Perphenazine-amitriptyline (Triavil)	Highly anticholinergic, sedating, and cause orthostatic hypotension Avoid in older adults with high risk of delirium, falls, and constipation
Skeletal muscle relaxants	
Carisoprodol (Soma) Chlorzoxazone (Lorzone) Cyclebenzaprine (Flexeril) Metaxalone (Skelaxin) Methocarbamol (Robaxin) Orphenadrine (Norflex)	Highly anticholinergic, sedating, and increase risk of fracture

Abbreviations: CNS, central nervous system; COX, cyclooxygenase; GI, gastrointestinal; NSAID, nonsteroidal anti-inflammatory drug; SR, sustained release.

From American Geriatrics Society 2012 Beers Criteria Update Expert Panel. AGS updated Beers Criteria for potentially inappropriate medication use in older adults. J Am Geriatr Soc 2012;60:619–22; with permission.

Rehabilitation therapies for older adults focus on optimizing functional status and reducing the risk of falls through the application of exercise programs, fittings for assistive devices, and other physical and occupational evaluations.[38,39] Pain relief using alternative movement-based approaches (eg, tai chi, yoga, exercise) and other non-pharmacologic approaches (massage, transcutaneous electrical nerve stimulation, acupuncture) has minimal safety issues for older adults, although levels of evidence vary among particular techniques.[29]

The management of chronic pain in older adults would be incomplete without recognizing the critical role of psychological therapies. Symptoms of chronic pain and

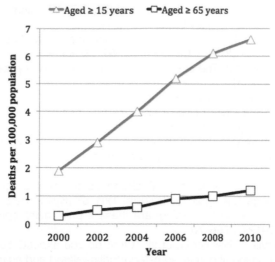

Fig. 3. Drug-poisoning deaths involving opioid analgesics. Deaths per 100,000 population by year from 2000 to 2010. Death rates for individuals aged 15 years and older and 65 years and older are represented by triangles and squares, respectively. Drug-poisoning deaths with the drug type unspecified (up to 25% of total drug poisoning deaths) are not included. Rates are age adjusted. (*Data from* Health, United States. Centers for Disease Control and Prevention. 2013. Available at: http://www.cdc.gov/nchs/hus/contents2013.htm; and the National Vital Statistics System, 2015. Accessed February 28, 2015.)

depression overlap closely and may be difficult to distinguish with advancing age, considering that evaluation may be more difficult in the presence of cognitive impairment.[25] Tools such as the Geriatric Depression Scale discriminate among older adults with and without low back pain.[40] However, older adults with chronic pain are less likely to use mental health services despite a similarly high prevalence of mental disorders as younger adults.[41] Additional research regarding effective ways to increase the prevalence of older adults that engage in psychological therapies such as cognitive-behavioral therapy, relaxation techniques, and biofeedback is needed.[42] Finally, effective pain treatments in older adults should also use community-based and family-based support systems (eg, preventive measures) that extend beyond the extent of pharmacologic and nonpharmacologic modalities.

SUMMARY

To effectively address chronic pain in later life, a multimodal approach to treatment must involve a meaningful assessment of pain in the older adult, an understanding of the patient's goals of therapy, and management including pharmacologic and non-pharmacologic treatments that incorporate the functional, cognitive, and comorbidity status of the patient. Because older adults demonstrate substantial heterogeneity with increasing age, treatment plans for chronic pain must be individually tailored to account for age-related differences relevant to pain physiology, assessment, and management approaches in later life.

REFERENCES

1. Institute of Medicine. Relieving pain in America: a blueprint for transforming prevention, care, education, and research. Institute of Medicine (U.S.) Committee on

Advancing Pain Research, Care, and Education. Washington, DC: National Academies Press; 2011 [Key Papers].

2. Brattberg G, Parker MG, Thorslund M. A longitudinal study of pain: reported pain from middle age to old age. Clin J Pain 1997;13:144–9.

3. Helme RD, Gibson SJ. The epidemiology of pain in elderly people. Clin Geriatr Med 2001;17:417–31.

4. Patel KV, Guralnik JM, Dansie EJ, et al. Prevalence and impact of pain among older adults in the United States: findings from the 2011 National Health and Aging Trends Study. Pain 2013;154:2649–57.

5. St Sauver JL, Warner DO, Yawn BP, et al. Why patients visit their doctors: assessing the most prevalent conditions in a defined American population. Mayo Clin Proc 2013;88:56–67.

6. Abdulla A, Adams N, Bone M, et al. Guidance on the management of pain in older people. Age Ageing 2013;42(Suppl 1):i1–57 [Key Papers].

7. Thielke S, Sale J, Reid MC. Aging: are these 4 pain myths complicating care? J Fam Pract 2012;61:666–70.

8. Gignac M, Davis A, Hawker G, et al. "What do you expect? You're just getting older": a comparison of perceived osteoarthritis-related and aging-related health experiences in middle- and older-age adults. Arthritis Rheum 2006;55:905–12.

9. Notcutt W, Gibbs G. Inadequate pain management: myth, stigma and professional fear. Postgrad Med J 2010;86:453–8.

10. Lowsky DJ, Olshansky SJ, Bhattacharya J, et al. Heterogeneity in healthy aging. J Gerontol A Biol Sci Med Sci 2014;69:640–9.

11. Katz B. Pain in older adults: special considerations. In: Raja SN, Sommer CL, editors. Pain 2014: refresher courses, 15th World Congress on Pain. Seattle (WA): IASP Press; 2014. p. 365–72.

12. Gibson SJ, Farrell M. A review of age differences in the neurophysiology of nociception and the perceptual experience of pain. Clin J Pain 2004;20:227–39.

13. Karp JF, Shega JW, Morone NE, et al. Advances in understanding the mechanisms and management of persistent pain in older adults. Br J Anaesth 2008;101:111–20.

14. Gibson SJ. Pain and aging: the pain experience over the adult lifespan. In: Dostrovsky J, Carr D, Koltzenburg M, editors. Proceedings of the 10th World Congress on Pain. Seattle (WA): IASP Press; 2003. p. 767–90.

15. Riley JL, Cruz-Almeida Y, Glover TL, et al. Age and race effects on pain sensitivity and modulation among middle-aged and older adults. J Pain 2014;15:272–82.

16. Cole LJ, Farrell MJ, Gibson SJ, et al. Age-related differences in pain sensitivity and regional brain activity evoked by noxious pressure. Neurobiol Aging 2010; 31:494–503.

17. Hilton D, Iman N, Burke GJ, et al. Absence of abdominal pain in older persons with endoscopic ulcers: a prospective study. Am J Gastroenterol 2001;96:380–4.

18. Mehta RH, Rathore SS, Radford MJ, et al. Acute myocardial infarction in the elderly: differences by age. J Am Coll Cardiol 2001;38:736–41.

19. Riffin C, Suitor JJ, Reid MC, et al. Chronic pain and parent-child relations in later life: an important, but understudied issue. Fam Sci 2012;3(2):75–85.

20. Cornally N, McCarthy G. Chronic pain: the help-seeking behavior, attitudes, and beliefs of older adults living in the community. Pain Manag Nurs 2011;12:206–17.

21. Ferrell BA. Pain. In: Osterweil D, Bummel-Smith K, Beck JK, editors. Comprehensive geriatric assessment. New York: McGraw Hill; 2000. p. 381–97.

22. Park HJ, Jeon YH, Rho MH, et al. Incidental findings of the lumbar spine at MRI during herniated intervertebral disk disease evaluation. AJR Am J Roentgenol 2011;196:1151–5.

23. Suri P, Boyko EJ, Goldberg J, et al. Longitudinal associations between incident lumbar spine MRI findings and chronic low back pain or radicular symptoms: retrospective analysis of data from the longitudinal assessment of imaging and disability of the back (LAIDBACK). BMC Musculoskelet Disord 2014;15:152.
24. Weiner DK, Karp JF, Bernstein CD, et al. Pain medicine in older adults: how should it differ?. In: Deer TR, Seong MS, editors. Treatment of chronic pain by integrative approaches: the American Academy of pain medicine textbook on patient management. New York: Springer; 2015. p. 233–58.
25. Herr K. Pain in older adults: approach to assessment. In: Raja SN, Sommer CL, editors. Pain 2014: refresher courses, 15th World Congress on Pain. Seattle (WA): IASP Press; 2014. p. 341–52.
26. Hadjistavropoulos T, Herr K, Turk DC, et al. An interdisciplinary expert consensus statement on assessment of pain in older persons. Clin J Pain 2007;23(1 Suppl): S1–43 [Key Papers].
27. Buffum MD, Hutt E, Chang VT, et al. Cognitive impairment and pain management: review of issues and challenges. J Rehabil Res Dev 2007;44:315–30.
28. American Geriatrics Society Panel on Pharmacological Management of Persistent Pain in Older Persons. Pharmacological management of persistent pain in older persons. J Am Geriatr Soc 2009;57:1331–46 [Key Papers].
29. Makris UE, Abrams RC, Gurland B, et al. Management of persistent pain in the older patient: a clinical review. JAMA 2014;312:825–36 [Key Papers].
30. Dobscha SK, Corson K, Perrin NA, et al. Collaborative care for chronic pain in primary care: a cluster randomized trial. JAMA 2009;301:1242–52.
31. Kee WG, Middaugh SJ, Redpath S, et al. Age as a factor in admission to chronic pain rehabilitation. Clin J Pain 1998;14:121–8.
32. Wittink HM, Rogers WH, Lipman AG, et al. Older and younger adults in pain management programs in the United States: differences and similarities. Pain Med 2006;7:151–63.
33. American Geriatrics Society 2012 Beers Criteria Update Expert Panel. AGS updated Beers Criteria for potentially inappropriate medication use in older adults. J Am Geriatr Soc 2012;60:616–31 [Key Papers].
34. Mitchell SJ, Hilmer SN, McLachlan AJ. Clinical pharmacology of analgesics in old age and frailty. Rev Clin Gerontol 2009;19:103–18 [Key Papers].
35. Deer TR, Prager J, Levy R, et al. Polyanalgesic consensus conference 2012: recommendations for the management of pain by intrathecal (intraspinal) drug delivery: report of an interdisciplinary expert panel. Neuromodulation 2012;15:436–64.
36. Christo PJ, Li S, Gibson SJ, et al. Effective treatments for pain in the older patient. Curr Pain Headache Rep 2011;15:22–34.
37. Manchikanti L, Benyamin RM, Swicegood JR, et al. Assessment of practice patterns of perioperative management of antiplatelet and anticoagulant therapy in interventional pain management. Pain Physician 2012;15:E955–68.
38. Ehrenbrusthoff K, Ryan CG, Schofield PA, et al. Physical therapy management of older adults with chronic low back pain: a systematic review. J Pain Manag 2012; 5:317–30.
39. Hiyama Y, Yamada M, Kitagawa A, et al. A four-week walking exercise programme in patients with knee osteoarthritis improves the ability of dual-task performance: a randomized controlled trial. Clin Rehabil 2012;26:403–12.
40. Rudy TE, Weiner DK, Lieber SJ, et al. The impact of chronic low back pain on older adults: a comparative study of patients and controls. Pain 2007;131:293–301.

41. McGuire BE, Nicholas MK, Asghari A, et al. The effectiveness of psychological treatments for chronic pain in older adults: cautious optimism and an agenda for research. Curr Opin Psychiatry 2014;27:380–4.
42. Braden JB, Zhang L, Fan MY, et al. Mental health service use by older adults: the role of chronic pain. Am J Geriatr Psychiatry 2008;16:156–67.

Palliative Care for the Geriatric Anesthesiologist

Allen N. Gustin Jr, MD[a],*, Rebecca A. Aslakson, MD, PhD[b,c]

KEYWORDS

- Geriatrics • Palliative care • Hospice • Do not resuscitate • Ethical dilemma
- Palliative sedation • Physician-assisted suicide • Perioperative palliative care

KEY POINTS

- The geriatric population is increasing, the number of chronic conditions within the geriatric population is rising, the use of palliative care and hospice within geriatrics has dramatically risen, and patients with chronic illnesses and end-of-life issues will present to the operating room more frequently.
- Palliative care and hospice are complementary and improve the patient's and family's experience with chronic illness and end-of-life care, but differences exist.
- Palliative care is not just care for those at "end of life" but is appropriate for any patient at any age in any setting (including perioperative settings) with chronic health conditions.
- Do-not-resuscitate (DNR) orders should not be automatically rescinded in the perioperative setting, but rather, conversations should occur to establish alignment of the goals of care of the patient with goals of care of the anesthesia and the surgical procedure.
- For actively dying patients, refractory symptoms that do not respond to conventional therapies may require the addition of palliative sedation for management of severe patient distress and suffering.

INTRODUCTION

The American population is aging. The percentage of the population older than age 65 was 9% in 1960 and is projected to reach 20% by 2050.[1,2] With increases in life expectancy, the burden of serious illness among older adults has also increased with

Dr A.N. Gustin and Dr R.A. Aslakson have no financial or industrial relationships to disclose.
[a] Department of Anesthesiology, Stritch School of Medicine, Loyola University Medicine, 2160 South 1st Avenue, Building 103, Room-3102, Chicago, IL 60153, USA; [b] Department of Anesthesiology and Critical Care Medicine, Palliative Medicine Program at the Kimmel Comprehensive Cancer Center at Johns Hopkins, The Johns Hopkins School of Medicine, 1800 Orleans Street, Meyer 289, Baltimore, MD 21287, USA; [c] Department of Health, Behavior, and Society, The Johns Hopkins Bloomberg School of Public Health, 1800 Orleans Street, Meyer 289, Baltimore, MD 21287, USA
* Corresponding author. Department of Anesthesiology, Loyola University Medicine, 2160 South 1st Avenue, Building-103, Room-3102, Chicago, IL 60153.
E-mail address: allen.gustin@lumc.edu

Anesthesiology Clin 33 (2015) 591–605
http://dx.doi.org/10.1016/j.anclin.2015.05.013
1932-2275/15/$ – see front matter
anesthesiology.theclinics.com

two-thirds of patients greater than 65 years old having multiple chronic conditions.[3] Moreover, providing high-quality end-of-life care is challenging because of multiple factors, such as the increasing number of elderly patients, structural barriers to access of care for older patients, and a fragmented health care system.[4] In a 1997 report that evaluated end-of-life care in the United States, the Institute of Medicine described significant patient and family suffering related to end-of-life care and emphasized the need for improvements[4] (**Box 1**). In the last decade and a half, hospice use has doubled and palliative care has made improvements with the development of guidelines and quality measures for the care of geriatric patients with chronic and/or severe illness.[5,6] A follow-up Institute of Medicine report in 2014 revealed that more work is needed to improve the quality of care for patients at the end of life, recognizing that palliative care services are underused and are too frequently unavailable, and that current providers should seek out further training in palliative care–related skills[7] (see

---

Box 1
Institute of Medicine recommendations and challenges for providing quality end-of-life care in America

1997 Recommendations for End-of-Life Care

1. *Raise the Issue.* People should think about, talk about, and learn about decisions they may face, as they or those they love approach death.

2. *Raise Expectations.* Dying people and their families should expect good, dependable care. They should expect their beliefs and wishes to be respected.

3. *Do What We Know Helps.* Doctors, nurses, social workers, and others need to use what we already know to prevent and relive pain and other symptoms.

4. *Get Rid of Barriers to Good Care.* Doing this often requires support of lawmakers, voters, the media, and health care managers.

5. *Build Knowledge.* The National Institutes of Health and other public/private groups should work together to find out more about end-stage disease and end-of-life care.

2014 Challenges for Providing Quality End-of-Life Care in America

1. Increasing number of elderly Americans, including those with some combination of frailty, significant physical and cognitive disabilities, multiple chronic illnesses, and functional limitations.

2. Growing cultural diversity of the US population, which makes it ever more important for clinicians to approach all patients as individuals, without assumptions about the care choices they might make.

3. Structural barriers in access to care that disadvantage certain population groups.

4. A mismatch between the services patients and families need most and the services they can readily obtain.

5. Availability of palliative care services has not kept pace with the growing demand.

6. Wasteful and costly systemic problems, including perverse financial incentives, a fragmented care delivery system, time pressures that limit communication, and a lack of service coordination across programs.

7. The resulting unsustainable growth in costs of the current health care delivery system over the past several decades.

Data from Institute of Medicine. Approaching death: improving care at the end of life. Washington, DC: National Academic Press; 1997; and Institute of Medicine. Dying in America: improving quality and honoring individual preferences near the end of life. Washington, DC: National Academies Press; 2014.

Box 1). Palliative care approaches and skills benefit geriatric patients, their families, and their providers not only in the course of general care but also in the perioperative setting.

PALLIATIVE CARE

The term "palliative care" was first coined in 1975 by a Canadian physician, Dr Balfour Mount, who was introducing "hospice-like" services into Canadian hospitals[8]; since then the definition has evolved[7,9–12] **(Table 1)**. In brief, palliative care involves (1) aggressive and expert symptom management, (2) psychosocial support of the patient and family, and (3) careful discussion about the patient's goals of care for his or her medical treatments.

In working toward these three goals, palliative care focuses on providing patients and their families with relief from the symptoms, pain, and stress of serious illness — whatever the diagnosis and whatever the outcome. The ultimate goal is to improve the quality of life for the patient and the family. Palliative care can begin early in the course of treatment of any serious illness and may be delivered in several ways across the continuum of health care settings, including the home, nursing home, long-term acute-care facility, acute-care hospital, intensive care unit (ICU), perioperative setting, or outpatient clinic.[7] Palliative care should be available when life-prolonging therapy begins, after life-prolonging therapy is withheld or withdrawn, and even for the patient's family after the patient's death[10] **(Fig. 1)**. **Fig. 1**A depicts the traditional model of palliative care where a patient first receives life-prolonging therapy until it fails, then palliative care is provided. **Fig. 1**B depicts the overlapping model where palliative care gradually increases while the patient receives a gradual decrease in life-prolonging therapy. **Fig. 1**C depicts the integrated model where palliative medicine is delivered at the onset of the illness and concurrently along with life-prolonging therapy. The intensity of palliative care increases and decreases depending on the preferences of the patient and the family. **Fig. 1**D depicts the ICU individualized integrated model where the patient receives palliative care along with ICU care. In the ICU, hospice care is not integrated into critical care because, though palliative care can be provided concurrent to critical care, hospice cannot. One should note that life-prolonging care ends

Table 1 Definitions for palliative care	
World Health Organization, 1990	Active total care for the patient whose disease process is not responsive to cure.
World Health Organization, 1993	The study and management of patients with acute, progressive far advanced disease for whom the prognosis is limited and the focus of care is quality of life.
National Consensus Project, 2004	The prevention and relief of suffering and the support of the best possible quality of life for patients and the family regardless of the state of disease.
World Health Organization, 2007	Palliative care as a pathway to improve the quality of life for patients and families with palliation and relief of suffering.
Institute of Medicine, 2014	The care that provides relief from pain and other symptoms, supports quality of life, and focuses on patients with serious advanced illnesses and their families.
Center to Advance Palliative Care	The specialized medical care for patients with serious illness.

Data from Refs.[7,9–12]

594

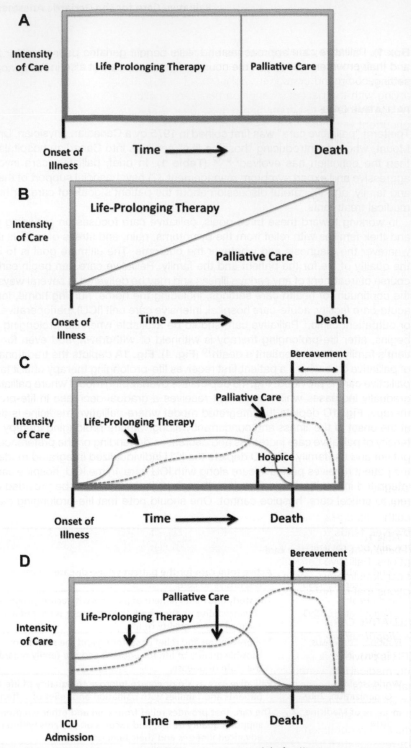

Fig. 1. (*A*) Traditional dichotomous model. (*B*) Overlapping model of palliative care. (*C, D*) Individualized integrated model of palliative care. (*Adapted from* Lanken PN, Terry PB, DeLisser HM, et al. An official American Thoracic Society clinical policy statement: palliative care for patients with respiratory diseases and critical illnesses. Am J Respir Crit Care Med 2008;177:914.)

at death, whereas palliative care peaks at death and continues after death to address the bereavement needs of the patients family.[10] Indeed, even in the ICU, expert statements recommend concurrent palliative and life-prolonging care with the emphasis varying with the patient's condition and care goals. Palliative care is appropriate at any age (pediatric to geriatric), at any stage in a serious illness, and can be provided concurrent with curative or life-prolonging therapies.[13]

Although palliative care is increasingly integrated into the continuance of geriatric care, it is still underused.[13] Despite national efforts to improve end-of-life care, proxy reports of pain and other alarming symptoms in the last year of life have increased over the last 10 years.[14] Moreover, advances in health care have transformed many previously lethal diseases (human immunodeficiency virus and AIDS, heart failure, chronic obstructive pulmonary disease, end-stage renal disease, and dementia) into chronic conditions with a frequent significant physical and psychological burden for patients and their families. To meet growing needs for palliative care, hospital, home-based, hospice-based, and community-based palliative care programs are increasing in number each year.[15] However, there are still not enough trained palliative care providers to meet demand; the Center to Advance Palliative Care highlights that there is approximately one cardiologist for every 71 patients experiencing a heart attack, one oncologist for every 141 newly diagnosed patients with cancer, and only one specialized palliative care physician for every 1200 persons living with serious or life-threatening illness.[10]

END-OF-LIFE CARE AND HOSPICE

End-of-life care refers generally to the process of addressing the medical, social, emotional, and spiritual needs of people who are nearing the end of life. End-of-life care may include a range of medical and social services, including disease-specific interventions and palliative and hospice care for those with advanced serious conditions who are near death.[7] More specific than palliative care, hospice is for dying patients. Although palliative care and hospice are complementary, differences do exist. Palliative care is based on patient and family need, whereas hospice care is based on patient prognosis. Palliative care can be provided with efforts related to restoring health regardless of any life-sustaining treatment (including ICU care). Hospice care, however, tends to focus on the patient's goals of care at the end of life and cannot typically be provided concurrent with aggressive curative or life-prolonging treatment options. Palliative care can be provided with no limitations to care—even with the use of cardiopulmonary resuscitation (CPR).[7] Hospice tends to discourage life-sustaining options that do not support the patient's goals of care.

PALLIATIVE CARE–RELATED PERIOPERATIVE ISSUES
Cardiopulmonary Resuscitation/Do-Not-Resuscitate Orders/Anesthesiology

CPR is provided approximately 800,000 times annually in the United States and is the only medical intervention for which no consent is required and where an explicit physician order is necessary for it to be withheld.[16] In 1983, the President's Commission for the Study of Ethical Problems in Medicine clarified that patients had a right to expect CPR as the standard of care in all situations of cardiac arrest unless a patient's wish was clearly documented to have it withheld.[17] From the 1980s to 1991, patient's do-not-resuscitate (DNR) orders were routinely rescinded on entering the operating room because anesthesiologists and surgeons believed that routine anesthesia and surgical care in the operating room (eg, volume resuscitation and use of vasoactive medications) would be considered "resuscitation."[18,19] However, in the last two decades, opinions have evolved such that some patients and providers believe that DNR orders should only apply to CPR in the event of an actual cardiac arrest and all the medical treatment before cardiac arrest is not CPR (and so should not be affected by a DNR order).[20] Moreover, studies still support variation in practice concerning management of DNR orders for perioperative patients. In one study, anesthesiologists were twice as likely as either internists or surgeons to assume DNR patients would suspend their DNR order in the operating room and, compared with these other providers, were less likely to discuss the implication of a DNR order with their patients, more likely to refuse to provide care for DNR patients, and more likely to ignore a patient's DNR request even if the patient made wishes explicit after an informed discussion.[21]

The Patient Self Determination Act of 1990 established as US law that a patient's right to self-determination was the supreme standard in medical ethics, taking precedence over beneficence.[9,22] Because of this act, routine suspension of the DNR orders in the perioperative period is considered a violation of the patient's right of self-determination.[23–25] As a result, the American Society of Anesthesiologists' practice guidelines refute required rescission of a DNR during the perioperative period and instead support the "required reconsideration" of a patient's DNR status before proceeding with surgery.[26] In that discussion with a patient, the anesthesiologist or surgeon should address the patient's goals and values in the context of the anesthesia and the surgical procedure.[18] In our estimation, four possible outcomes of this DNR discussion exist (Box 2). Clinical care should be discussed with the patient while keeping the patient's goals of care as the centerpiece of the discussion. The health care team is not ensuring a particular outcome, but rather ensuring that care is designed around the patient's individual goals and values, and is medically consistent with standards of care.[18]

Based on the previous discussion, patients with DNR orders can have a portion or all of their DNR wishes maintained in the operating room and perioperative period. Managing patients with care limitations and/or end-of-life issues can be psychologically and ethically challenging for some health care providers. An anesthesiologist may be presented with a clinical situation where he or she feels ethically uncomfortable to provide intraoperative care for geriatric hospice or palliative care patients at the end of life. In those circumstances, the American Medical Association Code of Ethics states that clinicians should not be compelled to perform procedures they view as inconsistent with their personal values but should involve a second anesthesiologist who is willing to comanage the patient by performing the desired procedure.[27] Consistent with this guidance, the anesthesiologist can refuse to provide care for a patient when he or she has fundamental ethical concerns, but the

---

Box 2
Outcomes of discussions with perioperative patients with DNR orders

1. Maintain the DNR status unaltered.

2. Fully rescind the DNR status in the perioperative period.

3. Accept certain resuscitative measures but refuse others, with all changes being fully documented.

4. Elect to the anesthesiologist or surgeon the right to determine which interventions are appropriate and which are not in accordance with the patient's stated wishes.

Data from Margolis JO, McGrath BJ, Kussin PS, et al. Do not resuscitate (DNR) orders during surgery: ethical foundations for institutional policies in the united states. Anesthesia Analgesia 1995;80(4):806–9.

anesthesiologist cannot abandon the patient and is required to promptly find another anesthesiologist who would be willing to provide the care. Similar to management of other patients with care limitations (ie, Jehovah's witness patients who refuse blood transfusions), anesthesia care practices may wish to develop individual practice guidelines to support and facilitate care of patients who wish to maintain DNR orders throughout the perioperative period.

Noninvasive Ventilation

DNR and do-not-intubate decisions to limit active treatments are taken immediately on hospital admission to protect patients from interventions that both contradict their preferences and values and also which could deprive them from communication with their families, particularly during the last moments of their lives.[28] The problem is determining when the clinical practice of noninvasive ventilation (NIV) support may be appropriate or futile.[29] Indeed, some perioperative patients with treatment limitations may refuse endotracheal intubation outside the operating room but may accept NIV because it may forego intubation while potentially providing relief from suffering caused by some forms of dyspnea. Some caution that NIV may be inappropriate in the context of any end-stage disease because of an increased use of medical resources, prolongation of the dying process, and intensification of suffering.[30] Yet, NIV may be beneficial for patients with progressive dyspnea and the use of NIV should be tailored to each patient's situation and each patient's goals of care.

Hydration and Artificial Nutrition

Cultural and religious variations among patients can create conflict between goals of care and the concerns about hydration and artificial nutrition at the end of life. The American Academy of Hospice and Palliative Medicine (AAHPM) endorses the ethically and legally accepted view that artificial nutrition and hydration, whether delivered parenterally or though the gastrointestinal tract via a tube (including nasogastric tubes), is a medical intervention.[31] The AAHPM recognizes that some faiths and traditions may consider artificial nutrition and hydration as basic sustenance or as symbolic importance, apart from any measurable benefit or the patient's physical well-being. Such views should be explored, understood, and respected, in keeping with patient and family values, beliefs, and cultures.[31] Members of the Roman Catholic faith view the removal of artificial nutrition and hydration as passive euthanasia.[32] Family members can also feel distressed when nutrition is withheld because they may believe that the patient "is starving to death." Thus, there may be equally good, ethical, and valid reasons for patients, particularly at the end of life, to either pursue or not to pursue palliative hydration and artificial nutrition. Moreover, anesthesiologists may care for these patients in the operating room for placement of feeding tubes and other procedures for providing enteral nutrition. Consequently, involvement in these procedures typically is aided by careful discussion of care plans and goals with the entire clinician team as well as with the patient.

ONGOING CONTROVERSIES IN PALLIATIVE MEDICINE
Palliative Sedation, Physician-Assisted Suicide, and Euthanasia

The concept of palliative sedation was introduced in the literature in 1991 to describe the practice of drug-induced sedation for terminally ill patients for management of otherwise refractory symptoms leading to unmitigated patient suffering.[33] Critics claimed this sedation was "slow euthanasia" or mercy killing in disguise.[34] Recommendations, guidelines, and standards for the appropriate implementation have been issued by national and international organizations.[8] Supporters note palliative sedation to be "the intentional administration of sedative drugs in dosages and in combinations required to reduce the consciousness of a terminally ill patient as much as necessary to adequately relieve one or more refractory symptoms."[20] In contrast to physician-assisted suicide or euthanasia, the intent of palliative sedation is to relieve symptoms, not to end the patient's life[8]; the intent of actions is the crux of care. Palliative sedation has critical ethical and legal considerations that require a foundation of clear communications and treatment objectives among all stakeholders (patient, family, nurses, doctors, clergy, and others). The incidence of palliative sedation is difficult to estimate (ranges from <1% to 30%) given the wide variation in definitions.[35] Many groups advise that proportionality is a key concept for palliative sedation with the depth of sedation recommended to be proportional to the severity of the symptoms.[8]

The AAHPM consensus statement regarding palliative sedation recognizes that palliative care seeks to relieve suffering (pain and distress) associated with disease but that, unfortunately, not all symptoms associated with advanced illness can be controlled with pharmacologic or other interventions.[36] Palliative sedation is defined by the AAHPM as the use of sedative medication at least in part to reduce patient awareness of distressing symptoms that are insufficiently controlled by symptom-specific therapies. The level of sedation is proportionate to the patient's level of distress, and alertness is preserved as much as possible.[36] The AAHPM also defines "palliative sedation to unconsciousness." This occurs when the administration of sedation is to the point of unconsciousness and can be considered when less extreme sedation has not achieved sufficient relief of distressing symptoms. This practice is used only for the most severe, intractable suffering at the very end of life.[36]

Currently, the ethical debates support palliative sedation for the management and relief of refractory or intractable symptoms.[37,38] The key ethical features are (1) the clinician's intent to relieve suffering, (2) the degree of sedation being proportional to the severity of suffering, and (3) that the patient (or surrogate) should give informed consent.[39] The American Medical Association Statement on the End of Life Care states that patients should have "trustworthy assurances that physical and mental suffering will be carefully attended to and comfort measures intently secured."[40] Palliative sedation is legal in every state in the United States and has been supported by the US Supreme Court in *Vacco v Quill* (521 US 793; 1997) and *Washington v Glucksberg* (521 US 702; 1997).[41] Anesthesiologists may wish to familiarize themselves with the ethical issue of palliative sedation because the drugs used for this practice include common anesthetics, such as ketamine, propofol, or barbiturates, and because the use of these agents in some hospitals may be restricted to anesthesia practitioners.

INTEGRATING PALLIATIVE CARE AND PERIOPERATIVE CARE FOR OLDER ADULTS
Palliative Care and the Surgical Intensive Care Unit

As ICU survivors increase in number and are studied beyond their ICU stay, the burdens of survivorship are coming into clearer view.[42,43] A broad array of physical and psychological symptoms (along with impairments in function and cognition) continue to impair the quality of a patient's life during and after the ICU.[14] Patients may have functional and neurocognitive deficits after surviving an ICU admission.[44–49] Not only are the patients experiencing symptoms of survivorship, the family members of critically ill patients can exhibit signs of anxiety and depression, along with complicated grief and posttraumatic stress disorder.[44,45] A "post intensive care syndrome" has been described for patients and their family members.[42]

Many ICU patients are unable to participate in shared decision-making with the ICU team and decisions must be made instead by surrogates.[50,51] These discussions may be particularly difficult because surrogates may respond to interactions with ICU staff by focusing on details rather than the larger picture, relying on personal instincts or beliefs, and sometimes rejecting prognostic information.[52] The need for specialist palliative care consultation is sometimes justified. Indeed, members of the ICU team should provide basic palliative care at all times. However, given that ICU personnel do not follow patients outside of the unit, specialized palliative care involvement can aid in care continuity for these patients inside and outside of the ICU (through recovery, discharge, and at home).

Unique barriers may exist for implementation of palliative care in any ICU. These barriers include unrealistic expectations for intensive care therapies for the patient by the patient, family, or ICU clinician; misperception that palliative care and critical care are not complementary and concurrent approaches; conflation of palliative care with end-of-life or hospice care; concern the institution of palliative care will hasten death; competing demands on ICU clinician effort; no adequate reward for palliative care excellence; and failure to apply effective approaches for system or culture change to improve palliative care.[13] Despite these barriers, palliative care is increasingly accepted as an essential component of comprehensive care for critically ill patients, regardless of diagnosis or prognosis.[14]

Implementation of palliative care in a surgical ICU can be uniquely challenging. Some evidence suggests that surgeons may have an exaggerated sense of accountability for patient outcomes and thus tend to do everything possible to avoid patient death.[53] Surgeons may believe that they enter into a "covenantal" relationship with the patient (and by extension, the family) and that patients and their families may consciously or unconsciously cede decision-making to that surgeon, particularly related to goals of care.[53] In a national survey, many surgeons described conflict with intensive care physicians and ICU nurses with respect to appropriate goals of postoperative care.[54] Also, surgeons described difficulties in managing clinical aspects of poor outcomes, communicating with the family and the patient about such outcomes, and coping with their own discomfort about these outcomes.[53] Given the strong sense of responsibility for patient outcomes, surgeons may be resistant to integrated palliative care in the ICU and may require encouragement from other specialties (including anesthesiologists) to consider palliative care options for patient care.[13,55]

As the longer-term impact of intensive care on those surviving acute critical illness is increasingly documented, palliative care can help to prepare and support patients and families for challenges after ICU discharge.[13] Key quality markers for palliative care measures have been identified and implemented in the ICU. The Care and Communication Bundle was developed and tested as part of national performance improvement by the Voluntary Hospital Association. The bundle is triggered by time and involve identifying the medical decision-maker and resuscitation status before Day 2 in the ICU, offering social work and spiritual care support before Day 4, and conducting an interdisciplinary family meeting not later than Day 5.[56] Anesthesiologists can advocate for more engagement of palliative care services for perioperative patients within the surgical ICUs of their institutions.

Palliative Care Consultation and Mechanical Circulatory Support Devices

Mechanical circulatory support (MCS) for patients with advanced heart failure refractory to medical therapy has made tremendous progress in the past 15 years.[57] Thousands of patients have had MCS devices inserted successfully as improvements in patient selection, surgical technique, and postoperative management have occurred.[57] MCS devices broadly include devices implanted to improve cardiac output on a temporary basis (extracorporeal membrane oxygenation) or for longer periods of support (the left ventricular assist device being the most common).[58–60] Compared with medical therapy alone, the placement of an MCS device improves survival, quality of life, and functional status in appropriately selected patients with advanced heart disease.[61] For a subset of patients with advanced heart failure, MCS device placement can be performed until a heart transplant is available (referred to as a "bridge to transplant").[57] Some patients may recover their heart function without ever needing a heart transplant (ie, recovery from viral myocarditis or postpartum cardiomyopathy) where the MSC device can be successfully explanted without further issue (referred to as "bridge to recovery").[57] For patients who are ineligible for cardiac transplantation (patient preference, age, or comorbidities), an MSC device can be placed with the intent that the device will remain in place for the duration of the patient's life (referred to as "destination therapy").[57]

Because MSC devices are now used more and more as destination therapy, placement is no longer restricted to the supply of transplantable hearts. Moreover, destination therapy adds particular complexity to the patient's treatment options and decision-making during the course of the MSC device as the patient approaches the end of life.[57] Several analyses have concluded that, in patients with an MSC device for destination therapy, the patients' goals of care often are undefined.[62,63] Without clearly defined goals or advanced directives, destination therapy may merely maintain circulation in a moribund patient, a situation sometimes glibly referred to as "destination nowhere."[64] Although the continuous-flow devices (ie, Heart Mate II or Heart Ware) have shown improved morbidity and mortality, hospitalizations are still frequent for bleeding episodes (usually gastrointestinal), arrhythmias, infections (especially of the driveline), respiratory failure, renal failure, right heart failure, and cerebrovascular events.[65] These adverse events may significantly affect a patient's morbidity and quality of life.[66,67] Because patients have the right to exercise autonomy, patients or family members may elect for deactivation of the MSC device if they believe that their goals of care are no longer achieved with the MSC device. Death related to deactivation of the MSC device is considered to be caused by heart failure, not from stopping the device.

Given these complexities, experts and practitioners have suggested that proactive perioperative palliative care may benefit patients considering MSC device placement and a study has shown feasibility of proactive palliative care in "preparedness planning" for MSC patients.[56,61,68] Indeed, the 2013 International Society for Heart and Lung Transplantation Guidelines published practice guidelines recommending specialist palliative care involvement in the care of patients being considered for an MCS device. The summary recommended that specialized palliative care be a component of the treatment of patients with end-stage heart failure during the evaluation phase for an MSC and that goals and preferences for end-of-life should be discussed with all patients receiving MCS as destination therapy.[57] In addition, the International Society for Heart and Lung Transplantation recommended that palliative care specialists be involved in the in-hospital management of all MSC patients.[57] Accordingly, anesthesiologists and the cardiac anesthesiologist should recognize greater involvement with palliative care specialists in the management of patients with MSC devices and can use these palliative care specialists more frequently when perioperative needs arise.

SUMMARY

Palliative care and hospice programs are expanding. Palliative care and hospice meet the physical, emotional, and spiritual needs of geriatric patients quite effectively, and have addressed many of the chief concerns voiced by those patients facing life-limiting illness.[69] Subsets of patients exist for whom conventional approaches to pain and symptom management by anesthesiologists and surgeons do not provide adequate comfort.[33] In these cases, immediate consultation with a palliative care specialist who has expertise in the management of these complicated patients and their symptoms is appropriate.[33] There is usually something that can be done safely, ethically, and legally that coincides with our duty to patient care.[33] Despite palliative medicine and hospice being in their infancy just a few decades ago, significant strides have been made. Palliative care and hospice have assisted in shifting the focus of patient care from a practitioner-centered and institution-centered practice toward a family-centered, patient-centered, and evidence-based practice.[7,21,70] Palliative care can provide aggressive symptom management in geriatric patients in the perioperative setting, even when patients choose curative or life-prolonging therapies.[18] For patients who are at the end of life, palliative care and hospice can allow the patient to die in peace rather than in a piecemeal fashion.[32] For those who are not at the end of life, this approach to patient care offers the same hope: to live in peace, not piecemeal.[71] Palliative medicine is consistent with our duty as physicians to help cure, provide relief, and offer comfort. "Guérir quelquefois, soulager souvent, consoler toujours" (cure sometimes, relieve often, comfort always).

REFERENCES

1. He W, Sengupta M, Velkoff VA, et al. 65+ in the United States. 2005. Available at: http://www.census.gov/prod/2002pubs/censr-4.pdf. Accessed February 20, 2015.
2. Bureau of the Census. Projections of the population by age and sex for the United States: 2010 to 2050. 2008. Available at: http://www.census.gov/prod/2010pubs/p25-1138.pdf. Accessed February 20, 2015.
3. Centers for Disease Control and Prevention (CDC). The state of aging and health in America—2013. 2013. Available at: http://www.cdc.gov/features/agingandhealth/state_of_aging_and_health_ in_america_2013.pdf. Accessed February 20, 2015.
4. Institute of Medicine. Approaching death: improving care at the end of life. Washington, DC: National Academic Press; 1997.
5. Teno JM, Gozalo PL, Bynum JP, et al. Change in end-of-life care for Medicare beneficiaries: site of death, place of care, and health care transitions in 2000, 2005, and 2009. JAMA 2013;309:470–7.
6. NIH State-of-the-Science Conference Statement on improving end-of-life care. NIH Consens State Sci Statements 2004;21(3):1–26.
7. Institute of Medicine. Dying in America: improving quality and honoring individual preferences near the end of life. Washington, DC: National Academies Press; 2014.
8. ten Have H, Welie JV. Palliative sedation versus euthanasia: an ethical assessment. J Pain Symptom Manage 2014;47(1):123–36.
9. Mahler DA, Selecky PA, Harrod CG, et al. American College of Chest Physicians consensus statement on the management of dyspnea in patients with advanced lung or heart disease. Chest 2010;137(3):674–91.

10. Lanken PN, Terry PB, Delisser HM, et al. An official American Thoracic Society clinical policy statement: palliative care for patients with respiratory diseases and critical illnesses. Am J Respir Crit Care Med 2008;177(8):912–27.
11. World Health Organization. WHO Definition of Palliative Medicine. Available at: http://www.who.int/cancer/palliative/definition/en/. Accessed on February 20, 2015.
12. Center to Advance Palliative Care. What is palliative care? Available at: http://getpalliativecare.org/whatis/. Accessed February 20, 2015.
13. Aslakson RA, Curtis JR, Nelson JE. The changing role of palliative care in the ICU. Crit Care Med 2014;42:2418–28.
14. Singer AE, Meeker D, Teno JM, et al. Symptom trends in the last year of life from 1998 to 2010: a cohort study. Ann Intern Med 2015;162(3):175–83.
15. Center to Advance Palliative Care (CAPC) Hospice and Palliative Care. Available at: www.capc.org/topics/hospice-and-palliative-care/. Accessed February 20, 2015.
16. Rubulotta F, Rubulotta G. Cardiopulmonary resuscitation and ethics. Rev Bras Ter Intensiva 2013;25(4):265–9.
17. President's Commission of the study of ethical problems in medicine and biomedical and behavior research. Deciding to forgo life sustaining treatment: ethical, medical, and legal issues in treatment decisions. Washington, DC: Library of Congress; 1983.
18. Scott TH, Gavrin JR. Palliative surgery in the do not resuscitate patient: ethics and practical suggestions for management. Anesthesiol Clin 2012;30:1–12.
19. Clemency MV, Thompson NJ. "Do not resuscitate orders" (DNR) in the perioperative period—a comparison of the perspectives of anesthesiologists, internists, and surgeons. Anesth Analg 1994;78(4):651–8.
20. Knipe M, Hardman JG. Past, present, and future of 'do not attempt resuscitation' orders in the perioperative period. Br J Anaesth 2013;111(6):861–3.
21. Broeckaert B, Nunez Olarte JM. Sedation in palliative care: facts and concepts. In: ten Have H, Clark D, editors. The ethics of palliative care: European perspectives. Facing Death series. Berkshire (United Kingdom): Open University Press; 2002.
22. Panetta L. Omnibus budget conciliation act of 1990. United States House of Representatives; 1990.
23. Cohen CB, Cohen PJ. Do-not-resuscitate orders in the operating room. N Engl J Med 1991;325(26):1879–82.
24. Truog RD. "Do-not-resuscitate" orders during anesthesia and surgery. Anesthesiology 1991;74(3):606–8.
25. Walker RM. DNR in the OR. Resuscitation as an operative risk. JAMA 1991;266(17):2407–12.
26. American Society of Anesthesiologists. Available at: http://www.asahq.org/for-members/medica/for%20members/documents/Standards%20Guidelines %20stmts/ethical%20guidelines%20for%20the%20anesthesia%20care%20of%20patients.ashx. Accessed February 20, 2015.
27. AMA Council on Ethical and Judicial Affairs. Physician objection to treatment and individual patient discrimination. CEJA report 6-a-07. Chicago: AMAPress; 2007.
28. Azoulay E, Demoule A, Jaber S, et al. Palliative noninvasive ventilation in patients with acute respiratory failure. Intensive Care Med 2011;37(8):1250–7.
29. Carlucci A, Guerrieri A, Nava S. Palliative care in COPD patients: is it only an end-of-life issue? Eur Respir Rev 2012;21(126):347–54.

30. Curtis JR, Cook DJ, Sinuff T, et al. Noninvasive positive pressure ventilation in critical and palliative care setting: understanding the goals of therapy. Crit Care Med 2007;35(3):932–9.
31. American Academy of Hospice and Palliative Medicine. Consensus statement on artificial nutrition and hydration near the end of life. Available at: http://aahpm.org/positions/anh. Accessed February 20, 2015.
32. Brody H, Hermer LD, Scott LD, et al. Artificial nutrition and hydration: the evolution of ethics, evidence, and policy. J Gen Intern Med 2011;26(9):1053–8.
33. Enck RE. Drug-induced terminal sedation for symptom control. Am J Hosp Palliat Care 1991;8:3–5.
34. Claessens P, Menten J, Schotsman P, et al. Level of consciousness in dying patients. The role of of palliative sedation: a longitudinal prospective study. Am J Hosp Palliat Care 2012;29(3):195–200.
35. Fine PG. The evolving and important role of anesthesiology in palliative care. Anesth Analg 2005;100:183–8.
36. American Academy of Hospice and Palliative Medicine. Consensus statement on palliative sedation. Available at: http://aahpm.org/positions/palliative-sedation. Accessed February 20, 2015.
37. Carvalho TB, Rady MY, Verheijde JL, et al. Continuous deep sedation in end-of-life care: disentangling palliation from physician-assisted death. Am J Bioeth 2011;11(6):60–2.
38. Broeckaert B. Palliative sedation, physician-assisted suicide, and euthanasia: "same, same but different"? Am J Bioeth 2011;11(6):62–4.
39. Homsi J, Walsh D, Rivera N, et al. Symptom evaluation in palliative medicine: patient report vs. systematic assessment. Support Care Cancer 2006;14(5):444–53.
40. American Medical Association. AMA statement on end-of-life care. Available at: http://www.ama-assn.org/ama/pub/physician-resources/medical-ethics/about-ethics-group/ethics-resource-center/end-of-life-care/ama-statement-end-of-life-care.page? Accessed February 20, 2015.
41. Bruce SD, Hendrix CC, Gentry JH. Palliative sedation in end-of-life care. J Hosp Palliat Nurs 2006;8(6):320–7.
42. Needham DM, Davison J, Cohen H, et al. Improving long-term outcomes after discharge from intensive care unit: report from a stakeholders' conference. Crit Care Med 2012;40(2):502–9.
43. Stevens RD, Hart N, Heridge MS, editors. A textbook of post ICU medicine: the legacy of critical care. Oxford (United Kingdom): Oxford University Press; 2014.
44. Pochard F, Darmon M, Fassier T, et al. Symptoms of anxiety and depression in family members of intensive care unit patients before discharge or death. A prospective multicenter study. J Crit Care 2005;20(1):90–6.
45. Anderson WG, Arnold RM, Angus DC, et al. Posttraumatic stress and complicated grief in family members of patients in the intensive care unit. J Gen Intern Med 2008;23(11):1871–6.
46. Cox CE, Docherty SL, Brandon DH, et al. Surviving critical illness: acute respiratory distress syndrome as experienced by patients and their caregivers. Crit Care Med 2009;37(10):2701–8.
47. Herridge MS, Tansey CM, Matte A, et al. Functional disability 5 years after acute respiratory distress syndrome. N Engl J Med 2011;364(14):1293–304.
48. Adhikari NK, Tansey CM, McAndrews MP, et al. Self-reported depressive symptoms and memory complaints in survivors five years after ARDS. Chest 2011;140(6):1484–93.

49. Iwashyna TJ, Ely EW, Smith DM, et al. Long-term cognitive impairment and functional disability among survivors of sever sepsis. JAMA 2010;304(16):1787–94.
50. Nelson JE, Meier DE, Litke A, et al. The symptom burden of chronic critical illness. Crit Care Med 2004;32(7):1527–34.
51. Apatira L, Boyd EA, Malvar G, et al. Hope, truth, and preparing for death: Perspectives of surrogate decision makers. Ann Intern Med 2008;149:861–8.
52. Schenker Y, White DB, Crowley Matoka M, et al. "It hurts to know... and it helps": exploring how surrogates in the ICU cope with prognostic information. J Palliat Med 2013;16(3):243–9.
53. Buchman TG, Cassell J, Ray SE, et al. Who should manage the dying patient?: rescue, shame, and the surgical ICU dilemma. 2002. J Am Coll Surg 2002; 194(5):665–73.
54. Buchman TG. Surgeons and their patients near the end of life. Crit Care Med 2010;38:995–6.
55. Shander A, Gandhi N, Aslakson RA. Anesthesiologists and the quality of death. Anesth Analg 2014;118(4):695–7.
56. Nelson JE, Mulkerin CM, Adams LL, et al. Improving comfort and communication in the ICU: a practical new tool for palliative care performance measurement and feedback. Qual Saf Health Care 2006;15(4):264–71.
57. Feldman D, Pamboukian SV, Teuteberg JJ, et al. The 2013 international guidelines for heart and lung transplantation guidelines for mechanical circulatory support: executive summary. J Heart Lung Transplant 2013;32(2):157–87.
58. Swetz KM, Kamal AH, Matlock DD, et al. Preparedness planning before mechanical circulatory support: a "how to" guide for palliative medicine clinicians. J Pain Symptom Manage 2014;47(5):926–35.
59. Long JW, Healy AH, Rasmusson BY, et al. Improving outcomes with long-term "destination therapy" using left ventricular assist devices. J Thorac Cardiovasc Surg 2008;135(6):1353–60.
60. Park SJ, Tector A, Piccinoi W, et al. Left ventricular assist devices as destination therapy: a new look at survival. J Thorac Cardiovasc Surg 2005;129(1):9–17.
61. Lietz K, Long JW, Kfoury AG, et al. Outcomes of left ventricular assist device implantation as destination therapy in the post-REMATCH era: implications for patient selection. Circulation 2007;116(5):497–505.
62. Dudzinski DM. Ethics guidelines for destination therapy. Ann Thorac Surg 2006; 81(4):1185–8.
63. Swetz KM, Mueller PS, Ottenberg AL, et al. The use of advance directives among patients with left ventricular assist devices. Hosp Pract 2011;39(1):78–84.
64. Bramstedt KA. Destination nowhere: a potential dilemma with ventricular assist devices. ASAIO J 2008;54(1):1–2.
65. Slaughter MS, Roberts JG, Milano CA, et al. Advanced heart failure treated with continuous-flow left ventricular assist device. N Engl J Med 2009;361(23): 2241–51.
66. Rizzieri AG, Verheijde JL, Rady MY, et al. Ethical challenges with the left ventricular assist device as a destination therapy. Philos Ethics Humanit Med 2008;3(1):20.
67. Rose EA, Gelijns AC, Moskowitz AJ, et al. Long-term use of left ventricular assist devices for end-stage heart failure. N Engl J Med 2001;345(20):1435–43.
68. Swetz KM, Freeman MR, AbouEzzeddine OF, et al. Palliative medicine consultation for preparedness planning in patients receiving left ventricular assist devices as destination therapy. Mayo Clin Proc 2011;86(6):493–500.

69. McCusker M, Ceronsky L, Crone C, et al. Institute for Clinical Systems Improvement. Palliative Care for Adults. 2013.
70. Quill TE, Abernethy AP. Generalist plus specialist palliative care–creating a more sustainable model. N Engl J Med 2013;368(13):1173–5.
71. Dunn GP. Surgical palliative care: recent trends and developments. Anesthesiol Clin 2012;30(1):13–28.

Index

Note: Page numbers of article titles are in **boldface** type.

Anesthesiology Clin 33 (2015) 607–615
http://dx.doi.org/10.1016/S1932-2275(15)00083-X
1932-2275/15/$ – see front matter © 2015 Elsevier Inc. All rights reserved.
anesthesiology.theclinics.com

Moving?

Make sure your subscription moves with you!

To notify us of your new address, find your **Clinics Account Number** (located on your mailing label above your name), and contact customer service at:

Email: journalscustomerservice-usa@elsevier.com

800-654-2452 (subscribers in the U.S. & Canada)
314-447-8871 (subscribers outside of the U.S. & Canada)

Fax number: 314-447-8029

Elsevier Health Sciences Division
Subscription Customer Service
3251 Riverport Lane
Maryland Heights, MO 63043

Printed and bound by CPI Group (UK) Ltd, Croydon, CR0 4YY

03/10/2024

01040488-0018